NATURE'S REMEDIES

AN ILLUSTRATED GUIDE TO HEALING HERBS

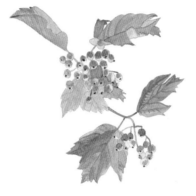

Jean Willoughby

Illustrations by Katie Shelly

CHRONICLE BOOKS

SAN FRANCISCO

Library of Congress Cataloging-in-Publication Data:

Names: Willoughby, Jean, author.
Title: Nature's remedies : an illustrated guide to healing herbs / Jean Willoughby ; illustrated by Katie Shelly.
Description: San Francisco : Chronicle Books, 2016. | Includes index.
Identifiers: LCCN 2016018842 | ISBN 9781452156026 (hardback)
Subjects: LCSH: Herbs—Therapeutic use. | Medicinal plants. | Alternative medicine. | BISAC: HEALTH & FITNESS / Herbal Medications. | MEDICAL / Alternative Medicine.
Classification: LCC RM666.H33 W55 2016 | DDC 615.3/21—dc23 LC record available at https://lccn.loc.gov/2016018842

Manufactured in China

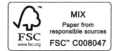

MIX
Paper from
responsible sources
FSC
www.fsc.org
FSC™ C008047

Design by Tandem Books

10 9 8 7 6 5 4 3 2 1

Chronicle Books LLC
680 Second Street
San Francisco, California 94107
www.chroniclebooks.com

CONTENTS

EMOTIONAL BALANCE & STRESS MANAGEMENT 61

HORMONAL HARMONY 81

MENTAL CLARITY & FOCUS 97

INTRODUCTION

Herbs delight our senses. If you've ever enjoyed a soothing cup of herbal tea or a well-seasoned meal, then you've already experienced a little of what herbs have to offer. Herbs add fragrance and flavor to foods and drinks like nothing else, but they are also powerfully effective in promoting health and well-being.

A medicinal herb is any plant that can be used to heal or nourish. Worldwide there are an estimated eighty thousand species of edible plants known to provide some aspect of this practical value. For this book, I selected more than sixty of the most well-known and effective medicinal herbs, most of which have played a vital role in the practice of traditional herbal medicine throughout history.

These easy-to-use herbs work exceptionally well for dozens of common ailments. Colds, stomach upsets, sleeplessness, fatigue, "the winter blues," headaches—these happen to all of us at some point. Learning about herbs can empower you with safe, natural ways to remedy these troubles while also improving your overall health. In this guide, you will learn about practical ways to use herbs in everyday life and gain a foundation of knowledge that will enable you to continue your exploration. You will read about the most widely recognized benefits of each herb and learn fascinating facts about how herbs work, how they are prepared, and the history of herbs as healing aids.

Herbs have beneficial properties and health-enhancing effects thanks to the impressive variety of nutrients and phytochemicals (chemicals naturally produced by plants) they contain. Peppermint, for example, contains the organic compound menthol, which produces a cooling sensation—contributing to an anti-inflammatory response—when it comes into contact with skin receptors in the mouth (as when we are drinking peppermint tea) or on our hands (as when applying a salve). Herbs are often categorized based upon these actions or properties and their affinities for healing and soothing certain areas of the body, such as the skin, sinuses, or digestive system.

To better understand the healing power of herbs, consider the heartiness of plants. Plants can't pull up their roots and leave when times get tough. They have to react and adapt to their surroundings. Plants survive and thrive thanks to an array of chemical compounds that they produce, many of which function to help protect them from environmental stress. It's thought that consuming many of the same compounds that fortify plants in turn enhances our own health.

Equal parts art and science, herbal medicine seeks to address the underlying factors that contribute to health and illness. In doing so, it aspires to improve our overall quality of life. As we all know, enhancing our health is not limited to treating everyday ailments or concerns. While herbs can no doubt serve as remarkably effective remedies for particular ailments, the goal of herbal medicine is broader: to promote robust health and radiant well-being. By learning about herbs—the vast majority of which are safe, affordable, accessible, and effective—we become better able to take care of each other and ourselves and attain a more resilient state of health.

It's no wonder that so many herbs have been thought of as "gifts from the gods" in cultures around the world. Herbs offer us not only trusted remedies, but also enjoyment as sources of beauty, pleasure, and creative fulfillment. After reading this book, you may even be inspired to grow a few of these little gifts of the earth at home. Wherever your desire to learn takes you, I hope you venture onward with excitement about herbs and how they can enrich your life.

A SHORT HISTORY OF HERBS

Herbs have been utilized and celebrated by almost every culture around the world. Their role in food and medicine is deeply rooted throughout human history. Archaeological studies suggest that herbs were consumed by our Paleolithic ancestors more than fifty thousand years ago. The earliest written works on plants and their use in medicine come from the ancient Sumerians and Egyptians, who began making lists of ailments and herbal remedies as early as 1700 B.C.E. Sumerian pharmacists wrote their herbal prescriptions in cuneiform—an ancient system of writing—on clay tablets. Egyptian medical papyri document dozens of herbs and their uses that are familiar to us today, such as aloe vera for soothing the skin, licorice root for coughs, and garlic and onions to help prevent colds.

In many parts of the world, indigenous and traditional knowledge of plants has been transformed into highly developed systems of medicine. In China, the use of herbs in healing goes back as early as the Shang dynasty, which arose in the sixteenth century B.C.E. In India, the Ayurvedic tradition reaches back more than three thousand years. In early texts from both traditions, we find catalogs of herbs and their uses along with intriguing philosophical ideas and doctrines about the nature of health and healing. Throughout the Americas and Africa, people developed rich and complex relationships with plants used in healing and spiritual practices, the knowledge of which was largely passed on through oral tradition and apprenticeships.

In the fifth century B.C.E., the healing properties of plants were promoted by the legendary Greek physician Hippocrates, regarded as the "father of Western medicine" for his enduring contributions to the study of health and illness. His teachings are expressed in the *Hippocratic Corpus*, a collection of some sixty tracts on the practice of medicine, attributed largely to his students. The *Corpus* is thought to be the first written work to provide a rational basis for understanding the functions of the human body and the origins of illness. Hippocrates and his followers advocated the use of medicinal plants and focused on the role of diet in healing. Later Greek physicians and botanists drew on the work of Hippocrates and earlier traditions to produce written herbals—collections of herbs described for their medicinal and culinary purposes—between the fourth and first centuries B.C.E.

Over time, an increasingly systematic approach to the classification of plants developed, as is evident in the work of Pedanius Dioscorides, a Greek physician and the author of *De Materia Medica*, a five-volume encyclopedia of herbal medicine written between the years 50 and 70 c.e. For more than fifteen hundred years, *De Materia Medica* was the most widely circulated and read text on herbal medicine. Containing detailed descriptions of about six hundred plants, it was to become part of the basis for the European pharmacopoeia and medieval medicine in the Islamic world, a foundational text for the science of botany, and an inspiration behind the creation of the great monastic herb gardens of the Middle Ages.

From the twelfth century onward, numerous herbals were published in Europe and the Americas. John Gerard's *Herball, or Generall Historie of Plantes* became the most-read herbal in English. Gerard drew heavily on the work of the Flemish botanist Rembert Dodoens, whose seven-hundred-page tome, *Cruydeboeck*, was reputed to be the most translated book after the Bible at the time. Nicholas Culpeper's *The English Physician* and *Complete Herbal* were published in the 1650s and not only proved enormously popular in their own time but have yet to go out of print. In Mexico, the first known herbal in the Americas was written and illustrated by two indigenous students in 1552. Their *Libellus de Medicinalibus Indorum Herbis*, Latin for "The Little Book of the Medicinal Herbs of the Indians," was originally written in Nāhuatl. The book depicts about two hundred herbs used by indigenous people and the elaborate classification system of the Nahuas.

The practice of traditional herbal medicine has also been a sphere of continual cultural exchange. In the

Americas in particular, numerous traditions have encountered one another. In the colonial era, African Americans relied upon medicinal plants for health care and developed remedies based upon practices exchanged with Native Americans and Europeans, as well as on knowledge of local plants and spiritual traditions. Over time, hundreds of native plants used by indigenous Americans have been added to the Western materia medica, a body of collective knowledge about herbs and other medicines. Throughout the mountain cultures of Appalachia (ranging from southern New York to northern Georgia), the interaction of Native American, African, English, Irish, Scottish, and German practices led to a diverse mixture of folk medicine traditions.

In the nineteenth century, many herbs were transformed into prescription drugs and sold in pharmacies. For the first time, through the advent of technology and chemical analysis, the active constituents in plants could be isolated and extracted. This contributed to the development of many new and potent medicines.

In English, we use the word *drug* broadly to describe medicines and other chemical substances. The word is thought to derive from earlier French and Dutch terms referring to dried plant material. This is fascinating because of how the word itself embodies the roots of modern medicine. Today, plant-derived ingredients are used in at least seven thousand medical compounds. In this, the world's herbal heritage continues to provide an endless source of aid and comfort, and reflects our reliance on nature to heal and make us well.

HOW TO USE
THIS BOOK

This book aims to show you how simple and enjoyable herbs can be, and to help you use herbal remedies easily and often. It is organized by the various benefits herbs offer to your health—for example, improved sleep, hormonal harmony, and emotional balance. Chapters include the most common ailments in each category and suggest a handful of trusted herbs—plus a few herb combinations—to help treat them. It's a succinct sampler, a tasting menu, a starter kit—something to orient you in the wide world of herbs. Here's what you'll learn about each of the more than sixty herbs presented in this book:

Common Name: An herb's common name refers to how it is known in everyday life. The common name might refer to its physical attributes or one of its benefits. Herbs often have a variety of common names, reflecting their places in the herbal traditions of different groups throughout history. The common herb names used in this book are the most widely used terms today.

Botanical Name: An herb's botanical name, which typically appears in Latin, is used for classification purposes, offering a standardized naming system that can be employed by scientists around the world.

Origins: Though often widely available today, many herbs were originally found only in their native regions, where they thrived because of local climatic conditions and soil types.

Description: Each herb in this book is accompanied by a paragraph that briefly describes its history, properties, and uses, as well as information about the parts of the plant that are typically used in herbal medicine and the beneficial nutrients and phytochemicals that they contain. (Refer to the Glossary, page 152, for definitions of herbal properties you'll encounter in these descriptions.)

Spotlight Herbs: In each chapter, you will also find an herb or a combination of herbs highlighted for their especially remarkable ability to heal and strengthen a particular body system. Each of these herbs is highly valued for its tonic properties—*tonic* referring to its ability to remedy imbalances in the body, prevent illness, and promote longevity. These sections explain the unique benefits of these herbal tonics and how they work to strengthen, tone, and reinvigorate different systems within the body.

PRACTICAL APPLICATIONS OF HERBS

There are many different ways to bring herbs into your life, from sipping soothing herbal teas to applying a salve to your skin. Depending on many factors, some herbs can be enjoyed in several different forms while others tend to be most effective in one form. Here are the forms you'll commonly find prepared by herbalists and marketed in herb stores and supermarkets. (Dosages and ingredients should be printed on the packaging. Read labels carefully to maximize benefits and avoid unpleasant reactions.)

Capsules: Capsules are very easy to take and contain either dried herbs or liquid herbal extracts that are encased in gelatin or a cellulose-based material. The cellulose used in capsules is typically taken from pine trees, whereas gelatin is an animal-based product. Easy to find in herb stores or supermarkets, capsules can vary in their strength due in part to the amount of herb (in milligrams) that they contain and what process was used to extract the active compounds of the herbs. For example, drying certain herbs can help concentrate their constituents, while other herbs are better suited to an extraction process that takes place when the herbs are still fresh.

Essential Oils: An essential oil, which can be applied topically, is a concentrated liquid that contains the aromatic compounds of a plant. These compounds are usually obtained through a distillation process, such as steam distillation, cold pressing, or solvent-based extraction. Essential oils are often referred to as "volatile oils," which partly refers to the fact that they are unstable and tend to dissipate quickly into the air at room temperature (unlike heavier, more stable oils like olive or almond oil). The most commonly used essential oils in aromatherapy, like lavender and rosemary, are steam distilled using hot water. Other distillation methods include cold pressing as well as solvent-based extraction, which relies on a chemical solvent such as alcohol to dissolve the plant material. Essential oils, which are commonly packaged in glass bottles, are often combined with carrier oils like olive, almond, or apricot kernel oil, or blended in very small amounts into herbal products like salves.

Herbal Oils: Herbal oils are typically not as concentrated as essential oils. Instead of using steam or solvent-based methods to distill the compounds, herbal oils are made by infusing herbs into oil using a double boiler on the stove or by relying on the sun to warm the herbs in the oil over the course of several weeks. Herbal oils may be applied topically on their own or used to make salves and creams.

Decoctions: A decoction is a drinkable liquid produced by simmering or boiling plant material in hot water over the course of an hour or more, which helps dissolve the plants' nutrients and phytochemicals into a rich drink or broth. Decoctions are similar to herbal infusions or teas in their use of hot water, but, unlike teas, decoctions are typically made with harder plant materials like roots, stems, bark, and seeds.

Infusions, or Teas: Herbal infusions—or "teas," as they are commonly known—are created by using water to dissolve the compounds of herbs. The herbs are steeped and then strained from the liquid and discarded, leaving behind a flavorful drink. Many herbs contain aromatic oils and other compounds that can be easily infused into a tea in minutes. Tea has the ability to warm, cool, and soothe like no other beverage, so it makes sense that herbalists would rely on herbal teas for helping to treat just about everything.

Liquid Extracts: Liquid extracts are concentrated formulas created by adding herbs to a solvent that extracts their various compounds. Makers of herbal products commonly use glycerin and carbon dioxide as solvents. Glycerin is a liquid produced from vegetable oils like coconut or soy. It can be easily purchased online or from health food stores and used to make your own herbal "glycerites." Liquid extracts are commonly packaged in glass bottles with dropper caps, and can be used either undiluted by placing drops directly on the tongue, or diluted by blending drops with another liquid. Using liquid carbon dioxide as a solvent produces another common type of liquid extract. This method is referred to as CO_2 extraction and is typically used by manufacturers to produce concentrated herbal formulas.

Tinctures: Tinctures, like liquid extracts, are applied directly to the tongue or blended with another liquid, and are created by suspending herbs in a solvent—specifically, alcohol. Alcohol helps dissolve plant material and extracts the herb's compounds, making them available for consumption. Alcohol works well for this purpose because it is both an edible and a preservative substance, which greatly helps increase the shelf life of the tincture and allows the compounds of the herb to be easily absorbed by the body.

Salves, Creams, and Poultices: Salves are created by concentrating and suspending herb compounds in a mixture of oil and wax, which enables them to be easily applied to the skin. When rubbed into the skin, salves can soothe aches and pains, sore muscles, bug bites, rashes, dryness, and inflammation. Creams are used much like salves and are generally made from similar ingredients. However, the ingredients typically include water and are processed by high-speed blending to create a whipped, emulsified mixture with the texture of lotion. Poultices are made from soft, moistened herbs that are spread onto a thin piece of cloth and then held in place on the skin. Salves, creams, and poultices are all ideal vehicles for herbal compounds that are most effective when applied directly to the skin. They are also among the simplest herbal preparations to make yourself and some of the easiest herbal remedies to use.

Syrups: Syrups are one of the tastiest ways to take herbal remedies. They work by concentrating plant compounds in water to which a sweetener has been added. Herbal syrups can be made using sugar or honey, but honey is often preferable because of its beneficial properties, including its ability to coat and soothe sore throats. Some syrups, like elderberry syrup, are made from single herbs, while others are made from combinations of herbs such as ginger, holy basil, peppermint, and chamomile.

Edible Plants and Culinary Uses: The benefits of many healing herbs can be enjoyed in everyday snacks and meals by eating the herb whole or incorporating it into a recipe. Many herbs have leaves or berries that can be consumed fresh or dried. These herbs may also be used as ingredients in foods and drinks, such as juices and wine. Examples of delicious herbal recipes abound, from using ginger and cayenne in stir-fries and sauces to adding lemon balm and mint to salads and smoothies.

STARTING OUT

If you're new to herbal medicine, start by trying out just a few herbal remedies. Have a cup of ginger or peppermint tea (pages 40 and 56) after one of your bigger meals during the day and notice how you feel afterward. Or, if you notice yourself feeling uptight or a little anxious, have a cup of holy basil tea (page 66) or take a dropperful of it as a tincture a few times during the day. Again, take note of how you're feeling.

Medicinal herbs work best when taken as part of a lifestyle that includes a healthy diet, daily exercise, and an overall commitment to self-care. While it's absolutely true that herbs can help you get back on your feet when you're feeling fatigued or stressed, they can't negate the long-term effects of consuming too many salty snacks or sugary, caffeine-laden drinks. (You have to kick those to the curb yourself.) But, hopefully, this book will help you replace some of your unhealthy habits (we all have a few) with herbs that strengthen your body and your resolve to treat your body better.

Another good thing to remember is that you don't have to limit yourself to herbal remedies to get your herbal medicine. You can cook with, eat, and drink your herbs too. Herbs liven up food like nothing else and add a healthy side of phytochemicals (mmm, right?) to your plate.

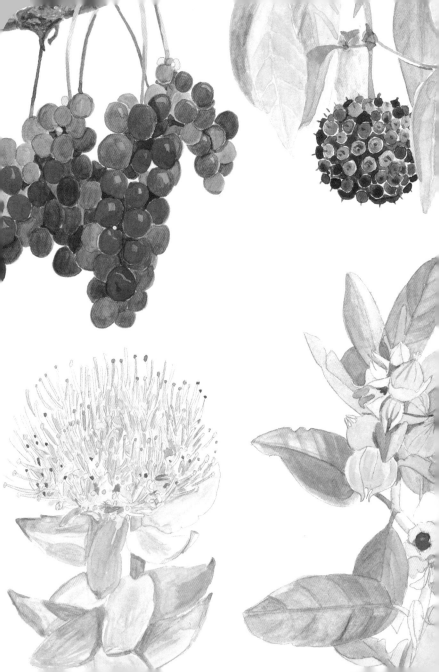

ENHANCED ENERGY

Everyday physical and mental stress sometimes makes us feel like our energy levels are running low. Travel, work, and major life changes can take a toll on how energetic we feel. When we have sufficient energy, however, we feel better equipped to handle our physical and mental responsibilities at work, home, or school. We can exercise regularly and recover from exertion easily. The world's earliest physicians, including Hippocrates, recognized that herbs can help us stay physically and mentally active, particularly during times of change or stress. Herbs contain powerful nutrients and compounds that nourish and energize, promoting a beneficial cycle of full activity during the day and restful sleep at night. The herbs highlighted in this chapter can help us fight fatigue, better adapt to stress, and improve our endurance.

ELEUTHERO

BOTANICAL NAME: *Eleutherococcus senticosus*
ORIGINS: Eastern Asia

Eleuthero appears in the earliest Chinese pharmaco-poeia, written more than eighteen hundred years ago. The celebrated sixteenth-century Chinese physician Li Shizhen wrote, "Holding a handful of eleuthero is better than having a cart full of gold and jade." The roots of the plant were valued in his day and continue to be used in herbal medicine today. Eleuthero is best known for its immunity-enhancing and "adaptogenic" properties. In fact, it was one of the first plants to be categorized as an adaptogen by students of the Russian physician Nikolai Lazarev, who coined the term in the 1940s to describe substances that safely help the body adapt to a broad range of stressors and generally enhance physical and mental performance. Eleuthero improves stamina and endurance as it gently increases energy levels. As such, it's an excellent remedy for fighting fatigue, particularly the feeling you may have when you have just come back from a big trip, gotten over a cold, or made it through a rough patch at school or work. It's also great to start taking in advance of stressful periods that you know are coming your way. Eleuthero is easy to find in cap-sules and tinctures, and the chopped, dried root can be prepared as a tea.

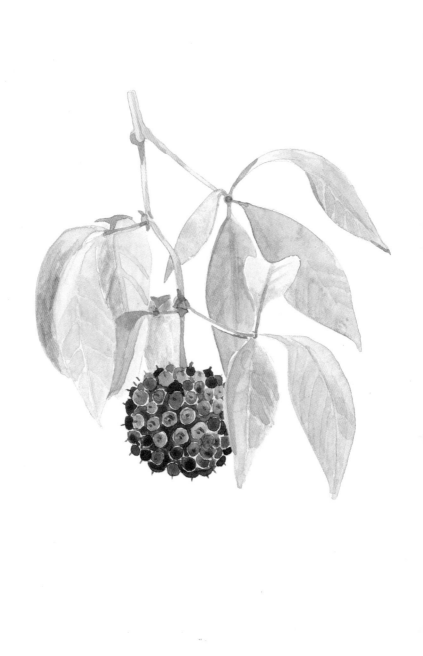

LYCIUM

BOTANICAL NAME: *Lycium barbarum*
ORIGINS: Southeastern Europe and Asia

Known commonly as "goji" or "wolfberry," the berries of the lycium shrub have been used in China and Tibet for thousands of years as a food and a medicine. They are thought to help energize and strengthen the body—from the immune system to the digestive system—thanks to a dense dose of nutrients. Just one ounce of the berries contains about 4 g of protein, 300 mg of potassium, and enough carotenoids— which are health-boosting nutrients—to give you 140 percent of your daily value of vitamin A. These carotenoids are joined by other phytonutrients (chemicals produced by plants) called flavonoids that have antioxidant properties and collectively give the berries their vibrant magenta-orange color. Herbalists recommend lycium to strengthen the eyes and skin, as well as major organs including the liver and kidneys. The dried berries have a mildly sweet and slightly salty taste. They can be purchased whole or powdered to add to smoothies, soups, and other dishes.

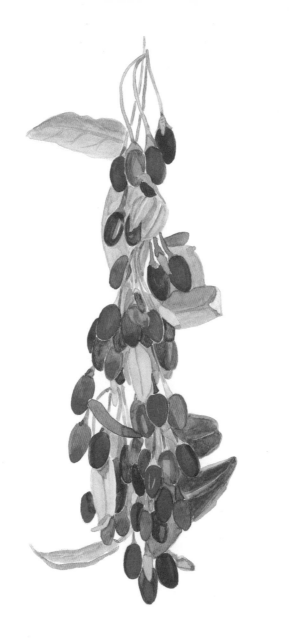

RHODIOLA

BOTANICAL NAME: *Rhodiola rosea*
ORIGINS: Europe, Asia, and North America

Rhodiola rosea—sometimes referred to as "golden root," thanks to its golden hue, or "rose root" for its rosy scent—has a long history of traditional use in Russia, China, Tibet, and Scandinavia. It grows in the wild in cold climates and mountainous regions throughout the Northern Hemisphere. The first-century Greek physician and botanist Dioscorides was the earliest to describe rhodiola in his herbal encyclopedia *De Materia Medica*, noting its use as a remedy for headaches. Today rhodiola is widely used as an adaptogenic herb to normalize bodily processes, including increasing physical endurance and stamina, reducing fatigue, and enhancing concentration. In addition to these uses, the contemporary use of rhodiola focuses on its ability to ease mild depression and anxiety. While there are multiple species that belong to the same genus as rhodiola and have been used in traditional medicine, rhodiola itself is the only one that contains rosavins, compounds that are thought to contribute to its antidepressant and antianxiety effects. Much like eleuthero root (page 22), rhodiola can be consumed in a capsule, tea, or tincture, and used to fight fatigue, stress, and a feeling of being run-down. It may also be combined with eleuthero and other adaptogenic herbs to help manage physical and mental stresses like extensive travel or challenging work schedules.

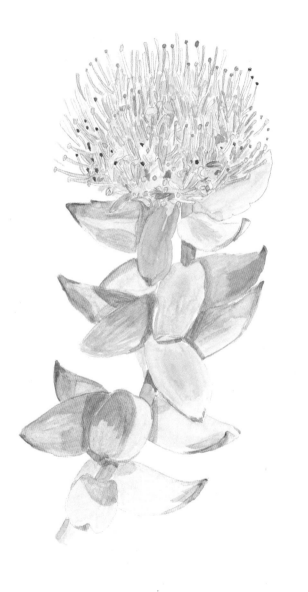

SCHISANDRA

{ **BOTANICAL NAME:** *Schisandra chinensis* }
ORIGINS: China and Russia

Schisandra is an adaptogenic herb that increases the body's ability to adapt to a range of physical and mental stressors. It appears to have gently stimulating effects on the immune, endocrine, and nervous systems, and is widely used to enhance stamina and concentration. Known as *wu wei zi* or "five-flavored fruit" in traditional Chinese medicine, schisandra is a storied herb with thousands of years of use as a food and a medicine to recommend it. First written about in the earliest Chinese pharmacopoeia, the *Shennong Bencaojing*, which translates into English as "The Divine Farmer's Herbal Classic," schisandra produces a rather unusual berry said to have five flavors: sweet, sour, and salty (flavors found in its flesh) and bitter and pungent (flavors found in its seed). According to tradition, these five flavors align with the five elements of nature: its sweetness with the earth, its sourness with wood, its saltiness with water, its bitter with fire, and its pungency with metal. The berries can be soaked in water and then strained to make a sour, peppery-tasting juice, but they are also commonly processed for consumption in capsules and tinctures.

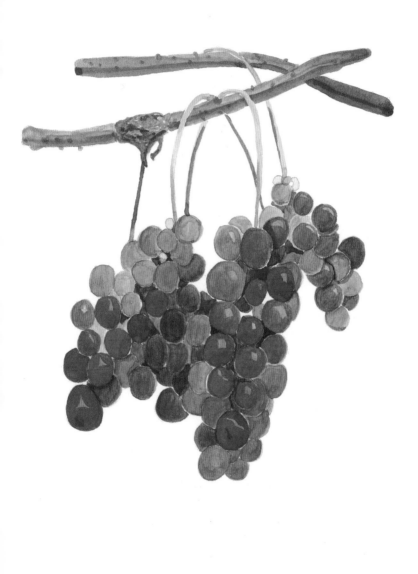

WITHANIA FOR
ENHANCED ENERGY

Withania, whose botanical name is *Withania somnifera*, has been used since at least 2000 B.C.E. in its native India and thrives in subtropical climates from North Africa to Nepal. Having both stimulating and calming properties, it is an extraordinary tonic herb for promoting enhanced energy and vitality. Its Latin species name, *somnifera*, means "sleep inducing" and refers to its ability to promote healthy sleep patterns. Because of its long history of use in India, the herb is also widely known by its Sanskrit name, *ashwagandha*, which refers to the scent of horses. Both the musky scent of the root and the rejuvenating effects of the herb were associated with the physical might of horses. In the Ayurvedic tradition of India, it is considered a *rasayana*, an herbal tonic that promotes health and longevity.

Withania is particularly remarkable for its abilities to support health and wellness in the young and the elderly. Because withania is a nourishing herb rich in iron, it's used to support healthy growth and development in children. Because it can help reduce the effects of aging on cognition and endurance, withania is useful for older adults. It also has anti-inflammatory properties that make it ideal for promoting convalescence after illness, injury, or overexertion. As an herb with antispasmodic properties, it can be used to alleviate muscle cramps and soreness following exercise.

Thanks to its combination of normalizing adaptogenic and calming nervine properties, withania is useful to people of all ages for promoting both physical stamina and mental clarity. It can help alleviate conditions that both stem from stress and contribute to it, such as nervousness, sleeplessness, and fatigue. Because it increases stamina, it may help promote greater physical activity during the daytime and more restful sleep at night. The powdered herb is typically combined with warm milk or water to make a drink, though withania is also commonly available in capsules and tinctures.

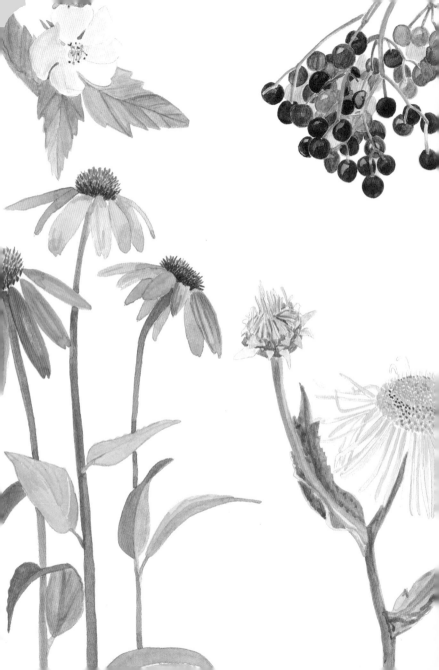

STRENGTHENED IMMUNITY & COLD RELIEF

When the inevitable seasonal cold afflicts us, herbs offer an assortment of time-tested remedies that can help clear congestion, soothe sore throats and swollen nasal passages, and reduce inflammation and fever—and some can even help prevent us from getting sick in the first place. Best of all, unlike pharmaceuticals, herbs don't cause unwelcome side effects such as drowsiness and cloudy thinking. The herbs highlighted in this chapter contain phytochemicals with antibacterial and antiviral properties, both of which may help reduce the duration of colds or act as preventative measures. Many of these herbs also stimulate the immune system, helping the body better cope with cold and flu season. This chapter illuminates the historical and modern uses of some of the most effective herbs in immunity and cold care and brings a few of our other herbal allies into the spotlight.

ECHINACEA

BOTANICAL NAME: *Echinacea purpurea*
ORIGINS: North America

Echinacea is native to central North America, and various species have been used for hundreds of years in many Native American communities as remedies for respiratory ailments and wounds. Following their lead, nineteenth-century American herbalists and physicians incorporated echinacea into formulas for treating colds, coughs, and infections. Today the large, stunning flowers of *Echinacea purpurea* are often used to add a spark of color to herb gardens. Here's a handy mnemonic to help you spot it growing: echinacea's scientific name comes partly from the Greek word for "hedgehog," *echinos*, which is what the spiny seed cone in its center resembles. While echinacea's flowers are quite photogenic, its roots have garnered far more attention. They contain antiviral and antibacterial compounds that are known to stimulate the immune system, inhibit inflammation, and reduce pain. (Please be aware, though, that individuals with autoimmune disease should avoid consuming echinacea.) In general, echinacea has been found to be most effective when taken as a preventative measure during cold and flu season or at the first sign of symptoms. Herbal tea blends and throat sprays made with echinacea may also help reduce the severity and duration of sore throats and coughs.

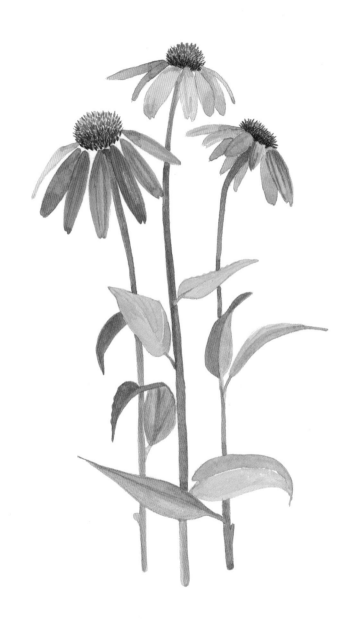

ELDERBERRY

BOTANICAL NAME: *Sambucus nigra*
ORIGINS: Europe and North America

Elderberry has been consumed across Europe and North America for thousands of years as both a culinary treat (enjoyed in the form of juice and wine) and a medicine. It has long been thought to enhance immunity and used to help treat infections. Native Americans employed various species of elderberry as remedies for colds, coughs, fevers, and sore throats. In traditional European medicine, the primary species used for treating these ailments was black elderberry, or *Sambucus nigra*, which is the most widely cultivated species today. Elderberry, which can be consumed daily in small amounts throughout cold and flu season, contains antioxidant and anti-inflammatory flavonoids and anthocyanins, which can help protect cells from damage. Other constituents include amino acids, potassium, iron, and vitamins A and C. It also contains B vitamins, notably thiamine, riboflavin, niacin, pantothenic acid, folate, and vitamin B_6. All of these nutrients make elderberry an excellent choice for jumpstarting your immune system. Elderberry syrup or jam is a great way to work the plant into your diet. It can be consumed daily in small amounts throughout cold and flu season. Elderberry juice can be enjoyed on its own, combined with other fruit juices, or used in winemaking to make a beloved traditional beverage for preserving the healing properties of the plant.

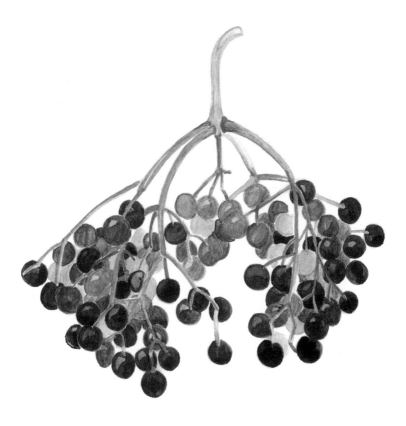

ELECAMPANE

BOTANICAL NAME: *Inula helenium*
ORIGINS: Central Asia, Southern Europe

Elecampane is an impressively large and long-stemmed flowering plant with a formidable root system. A member of the sunflower family, it's native to central Asia and southern Europe, and it has naturalized in North America. Its roots are used in herbal preparations for treating respiratory infections, coughs, and bronchial irritation. Considering that it can grow to between nine and ten feet tall, it may seem strange that elecampane was once known as "elfwort." The second half of the word, *wort*, comes from the Old English word for a plant or herb, *wyrt*, while the first half has a touch of magic to it. In early medieval England, elecampane developed a reputation among the Anglo-Saxons for affording protection from sickness, which they believed was caused by the machinations of spiteful elves—hence the moniker "elfwort." What they had right was that elecampane is indeed a powerful remedy for lung ailments. Its root contains essential oils and organic compounds with antibacterial and expectorant properties, compounds that are most effectively consumed in teas or tinctures. Elecampane soothes the irritation caused by bronchitis. It can also help reduce the severity and duration of coughs and lung infections. Elecampane even shows promise for treating some types of asthma.

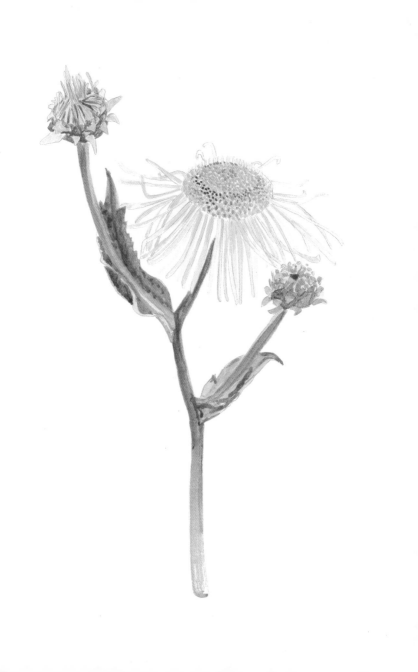

GINGER

BOTANICAL NAME: *Zingiber officinale*
ORIGINS: Tropical Asia

Ginger, a beloved and potent healing herb, was so highly valued in ancient times that it found its way into the Qur'an as a drink served in paradise. It was among the first herbs to travel the world as part of the emerging global spice trade in the ships of fifteenth-century merchants and explorers, who carried it from its native home in China to eastern Africa, where it still grows today. Perhaps more than any other herb, ginger is used throughout the world as a remedy for colds and flu. It has a piquant flavor that can be enjoyed in teas or as a culinary spice, and it exerts a warming effect when consumed. Its phytochemicals have antibacterial, antiviral, and antifungal properties. These compounds may work to inhibit rhinoviruses, the types of viruses that cause a common cold. Ginger is used both as a preventative measure and a fierce cold-fighter, treating all major symptoms: sinus inflammation, congestion, coughing, and sore throat. Its anti-inflammatory and pain-relieving compounds, called gingerols, help soothe achy muscles and may relieve some types of headaches. Ginger's spiciness and pungent aroma break through the cloud of congestion that hangs over everything when you're sick and can't smell or taste a thing. Ginger also acts as an antihistamine, which can help with allergies, motion sickness, and nausea.

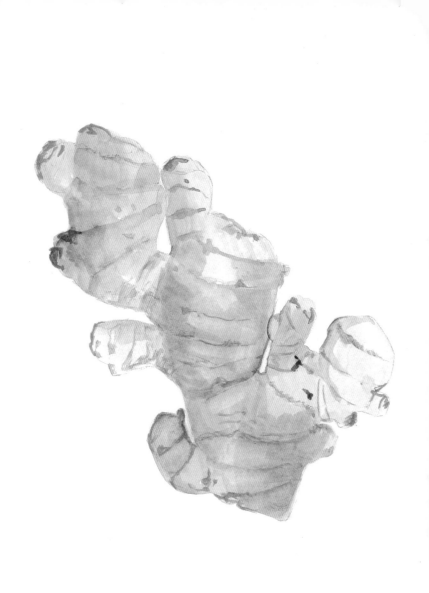

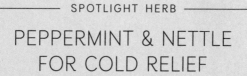

PEPPERMINT & NETTLE FOR COLD RELIEF

Healing herbs peppermint and nettle combine to make an excellent cold-fighting "pepper-nettle" tea that can be consumed throughout cold and flu season for cold prevention and as a remedy for cold symptoms. The two herbs are beneficial when paired together as they work to soothe inflammation in complementary ways. In particular, they share affinities for aiding the respiratory system and soothing irritated mucous membranes.

Peppermint (page 56), which is native to Europe and whose botanical name is *Mentha x piperita*, is cooling, both to the touch and to the taste buds. Even in full sun on a warm day, its leaves will feel slightly cool due to the presence of the compound menthol. Menthol is the active constituent in peppermint that helps to thin mucus and to reduce sinus and chest congestion. Peppermint also has antimicrobial properties, making it useful for getting over a cold or infection.

Nettle (*Urtica dioica*) is anything but cooling. Its fresh leaves are covered in fine hairs that seem to sting when they contact the skin, giving it its genus name from the Latin *urere*, meaning "to burn." When nettle is applied to an area of the body that is already experiencing pain, however, it works to reduce it. This effect comes from its ability to decrease inflammatory chemicals involved in sending pain signals to the brain. When nettle is processed, it completely loses its sting but retains its anti-inflammatory power. Nettle leaves are packed with nutrients, minerals, and phytochemicals that help boost the immune system. These compounds also help relieve irritated sinuses and lungs. The seventeenth-century English herbalist Nicholas Culpeper wrote that nettle leaves and roots were "safe and sure medicines to open the pipes and the passages of the lungs." Nettle remains popular today, especially in its native Europe and North America, as a remedy for respiratory ailments and as a culinary herb.

MARSHMALLOW ROOT

BOTANICAL NAME: *Althaea officinalis*
ORIGINS: Europe, Asia, and North Africa

Marshmallow root has been used in traditional medicine in Europe and India for thousands of years as a remedy for cold symptoms and gastrointestinal irritation. Today it is cultivated around the world as a perennial herb and used to treat a wide range of ailments. It's also the original source of the popular puffed confection by the same name. In nineteenth-century France, marshmallow root extract was whipped with egg white and sugar to produce a kind of meringue. This recipe is thought to have contributed to the creation of commercial marshmallows. Marshmallow root contains large quantities of mucilage, a gummy substance with demulcent properties that reduces inflammation of the body's mucous membranes by coating mucosal linings with a thin, smooth layer that helps protect them from further irritation. Marshmallow root teas and tinctures are especially helpful for treating dry coughs and soothing sore or dry throats. They also relieve irritation in the body's gastric and urinary linings, as well as in areas where the skin and mucous membranes meet, such as in the ears and nose.

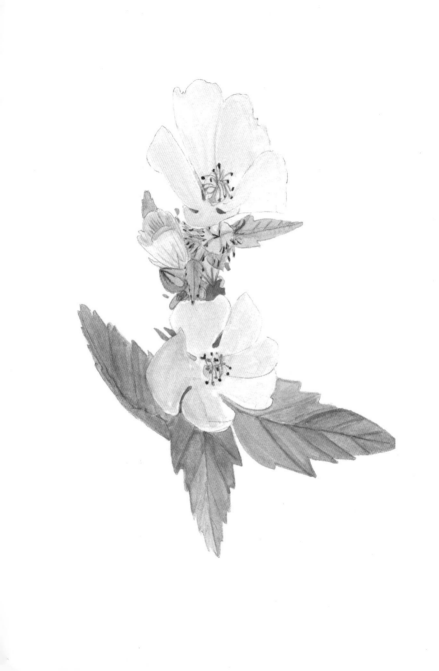

YARROW

BOTANICAL NAME: *Achillea millefolium*
ORIGINS: Asia and Europe

Cultivated varieties of yarrow are often planted in herb gardens, where their flowers bloom in shades of bright red and yellow. However, the best medicinal varieties are usually wild and produce chalk-white flowers, though truly wild yarrow can range from pale yellow to light pink. Yarrow flowers have a long history of use in many cultures and produce potent teas and tinctures that can alleviate a range of ailments. Native Americans from east to west used yarrow to treat pain and infections. Many tribes in the Great Plains region of the United States used yarrow specifically for earaches, headaches, and fevers. Today it remains a popular medicinal herb thanks to its versatility and effectiveness in treating many common ailments, from bruises and cuts to cramps and colds. It also appears to have a normalizing effect on circulation. This property, combined with its sweat-inducing capacity, make it a remedy for treating some types of fevers. Yarrow also contains antiseptic and anti-inflammatory compounds that may help reduce the duration of colds.

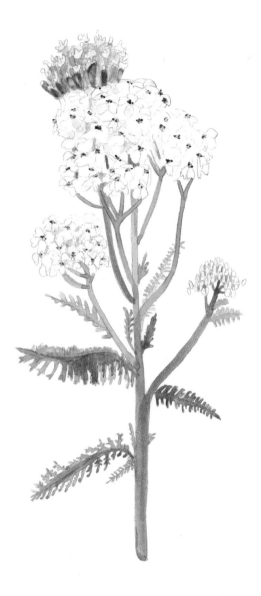

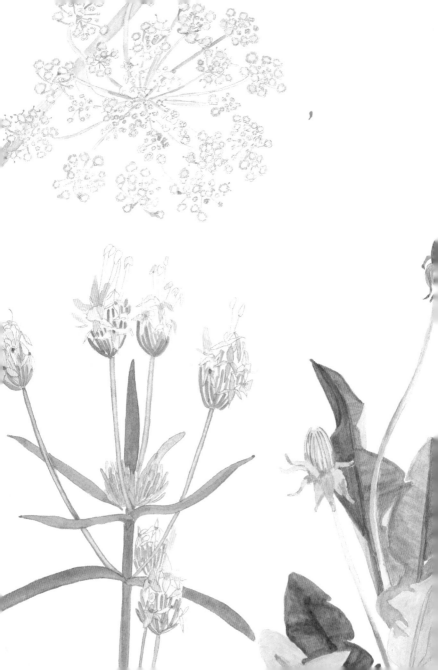

DIGESTIVE HEALTH

Digestive health is crucial to physical and mental well-being. Our digestive system—which is responsible for breaking down our food, absorbing nutrients, and expelling waste—is an elaborate, sensitive system of many moving parts and subsystems, one of which is the enteric nervous system, which runs the length of the gastrointestinal tract. Often referred to as the body's "second brain," it produces chemical helpers that regulate digestion. For example, serotonin, a neurotransmitter widely considered to contribute to feelings of comfort and happiness, is produced primarily in the gastrointestinal tract and plays a major role in regulating bowel motility. Despite having a second brain to coordinate activities, digestion is not always a smooth process, and discomforts are common. As we all know, it's an operation that can use a little extra help sometimes. The herbs in this chapter—many of which, fittingly, are also consumed for their flavor and nutritional value—are reliable and time-tested aids for improving digestion and relieving a range of digestive ailments.

DANDELION

BOTANICAL NAME: *Taraxacum officinale*
ORIGINS: Asia and Europe

Dandelion is one of the most nutritious and medicinally valuable weeds in the world. As gardeners and lawn-abiding citizens can attest, it reproduces prolifically and is difficult to uproot. It clings to the soil with a strong taproot, which is one of the parts used in herbal medicine. Its soft, silvery seed heads are the delight of children, who shake or blow on them, causing them to disperse and sow the next generation of tufted playthings. The name *dandelion* comes from the French *dent de lion*, or "lion's tooth," which refers to the jagged edges of the herb's long, slender leaves. As a bitter herb, dandelion stimulates the appetite and digestive system. It then enhances the digestive process by promoting optimal liver function. It increases the flow of bile from the gallbladder into the small intestine, which stimulates peristalsis, a series of wave-like muscle contractions that move food through the digestive tract. This contributes to dandelion's gentle laxative effect. It is also a diuretic, a medicine that increases elimination. As an edible wild food, dandelion is valued for its vitamin and mineral content. It contains significant amounts of B vitamins, as well as vitamins A, C, and E, and it's high in potassium, calcium, iron, magnesium, and manganese.

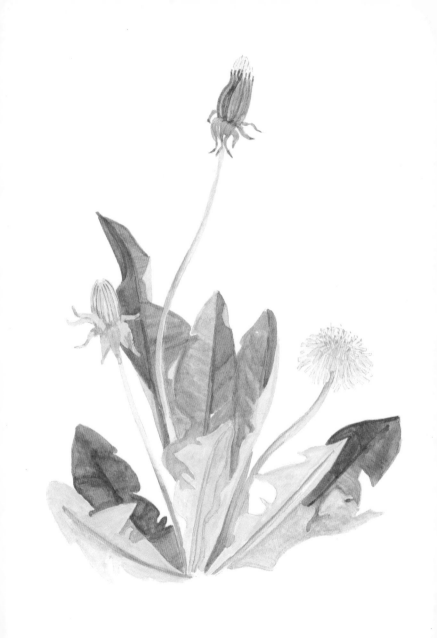

FENNEL

BOTANICAL NAME: *Foeniculum vulgare*
ORIGINS: Mediterranean Region

Fennel is an aromatic herb in the Umbelliferae family, named for the umbrella-like shape of its flowers, called *umbels*. It has been cultivated in gardens and used in cookery for thousands of years across its native range and beyond. The gifted twelfth-century German naturalist, nun, and polymath Hildegard von Bingen was among the first to praise fennel for its multitude of uses. In her medical treatise, *Physica*, she wrote that "in whatever way it is eaten, it makes a person happy . . . and makes his digestion good." Fennel has a unique, sweet-smelling fragrance and a flavor reminiscent of licorice and anise. Its seeds and leaves are used for improving digestion, and it contains vitamins A, C, and folate, as well as calcium, iron, and potassium. Along with these nutrients, it contains phytochemicals with significant antioxidant, anti-inflammatory, and anti-spasmodic activity. It soothes the stomach and acts as a carminative, a medicine that reduces gas. Fennel is especially helpful for soothing the feeling of bloating that comes from eating a heavy meal. In many areas of India and Pakistan, fennel seeds are often offered after meals as *mukhwas*, a sweet snack that acts as a digestive aid and breath freshener.

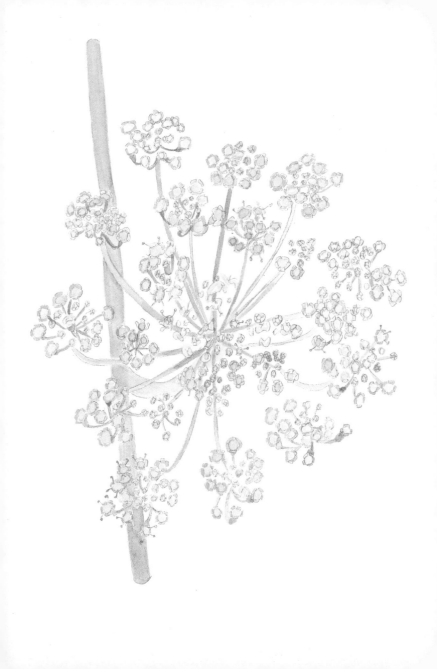

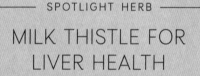

MILK THISTLE FOR LIVER HEALTH

Your hard-working liver is involved in hundreds of bodily processes. It helps break down the food you eat; removes toxins from your body; converts protein, fats, and carbs into energy and nutrients; detoxifies chemicals; and filters your blood. It even helps metabolize and regulate estrogen and testosterone, two of the body's primary sex hormones. It follows that a healthy, well-functioning liver is one of the body's best defenses.

Milk thistle (*Silybum marianum*) is one of the best-known plants used to protect and strengthen the liver. Native to the Mediterranean, milk thistle has been used for more than two thousand years to promote liver function and digestive health. Its common name refers to the milky fluid produced by the plant when its leaves or stem are cut or crushed. It is the seeds of the plant, however, that contain the polyphenol compounds called flavonoids that are considered to be responsible for milk thistle's medicinal effects. The seeds are processed to make capsules, tinctures, and liquid extracts.

Milk thistle helps the liver in three key ways. First, it helps regenerate liver cells that have been damaged by oxidative stress due to smoking, alcohol, medications, or exposure to toxins. Second, it protects liver cells by altering their surrounding membranes to prevent toxins from entering or causing damage. Third, it stimulates the production of new liver cells and contributes to the regrowth of liver tissue.

The compounds responsible for milk thistle's protective and regenerative powers are part of a flavonoid group called silymarin. This group includes compounds with antioxidant and antiviral properties. Silymarin is known to increase concentrations of glutathione, an antioxidant that plays an important role in ridding the body of toxins. It also contains sulfur compounds that scavenge free radicals and bind to toxins and metals, helping to safely remove them from the body.

PEPPERMINT

BOTANICAL NAME: *Mentha x piperita*
ORIGINS: Europe

Named for its pleasantly piquant aroma, peppermint is thought to be a natural hybrid of spearmint and watermint. The first specimens were described in 1696 by English botanist John Ray. It was added to the *London Pharmacopoeia* in 1721. Recognized for its many benefits and enjoyable flavor, peppermint was being grown commercially by the end of the eighteenth century. Though peppermint is a relative newcomer, other mint varieties have thousands of years of use to recommend them. The *Ebers Papyrus*, an ancient Egyptian medical text, lists mint as a remedy for upset stomach. Today peppermint is recognized as a premier digestive herb and is widely used for treating upset stomach, nausea, and indigestion. Its essential oil contains a high amount of menthol, which works to relax the muscles in the walls of the stomach and intestines. This makes peppermint an ideal remedy for soothing menstrual cramps, bloating, and gas. Menthol has a cooling effect, as it activates cold-sensitive receptors in the skin and mucosa. Peppermint also has antimicrobial properties and is a good source of manganese, copper, and vitamin C. The leaves and flowering tops are used in cooking, confectionery, and herbal medicine.

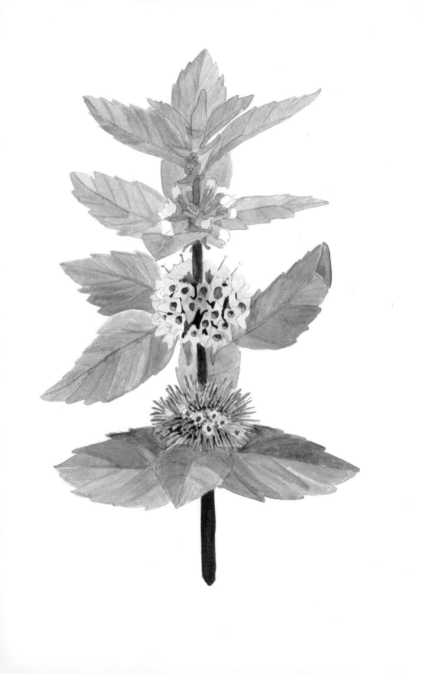

PSYLLIUM

BOTANICAL NAME: *Plantago ovata*
ORIGINS: Asia and Middle East

Psyllium has been cultivated for its medicinal value for thousands of years across southern and western Asia. Along with its close relative plantain (page 134), psyllium belongs to the genus *Plantago*. The term *psyllium* is used to refer to several plants whose seeds are used medicinally. Psyllium seed is valued for its high dietary fiber and mucilage content—mucilage being a substance with demulcent properties that relieve irritation by coating the body's gastric and urinary linings with a protective film. The mucilage in psyllium is concentrated in its seed coat. When being processed for medicinal use, this outer layer, or husk, of the seed is milled to a flaky or powdery consistency. The husks of *Plantago ovata* and its cousin *Plantago psyllium* are the primary kinds used in dietary fiber supplements. Dietary fiber is not absorbed by the small intestine but continues through the large intestine, softening and adding bulk to the stool. It absorbs excess water and stimulates bowel motility, resulting in a laxative action, making it a remedy for constipation. In commercial formulas, psyllium is sometimes combined with other demulcent and laxative herbs to soothe the gastrointestinal tract and promote regularity.

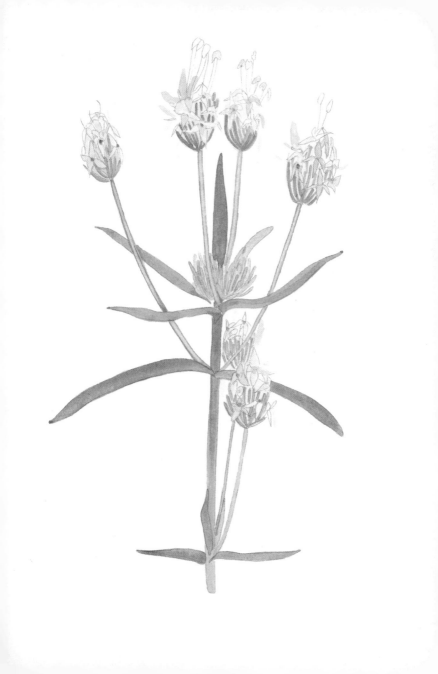

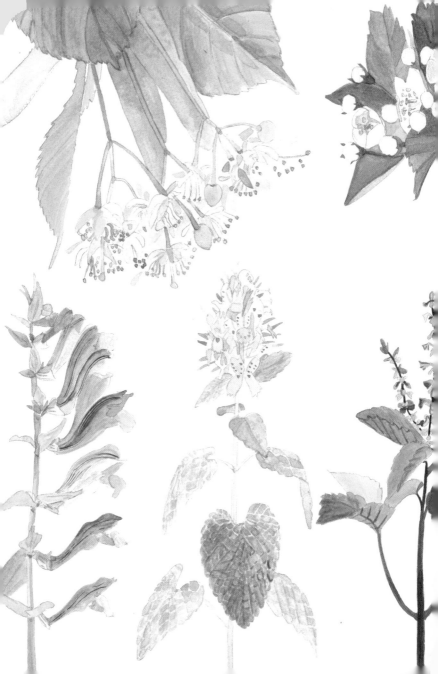

EMOTIONAL BALANCE & STRESS MANAGEMENT

Gentle, effective, and safe, herbs provide us with some of the most popular remedies for managing stress and emotions. Indeed, using herbs to relieve stress and promote emotional balance is a common entry point to the world of herbal medicine. Life can be stressful, and it's often challenging to balance the demands of work and home with our own needs. Such problems are, of course, not new. For thousands of years, people have turned to soothing herbs like skullcap, lemon balm, and lavender for their abilities to treat many of the same difficulties that we encounter today. As you'll discover in the chapter ahead, our ancestors learned about and adopted an impressive variety of herbs to calm the nervous system and restore emotional equilibrium. The herbs in this chapter are acclaimed for having these calming and uplifting effects on mood, as well as for their ability to alleviate mild anxiety and tension.

CATNIP

BOTANICAL NAME: *Nepeta cataria*
ORIGINS: Europe, Middle East, and
Central Asia

Catnip is one of the most eye-catching members of the mint family, with heart-shaped leaves that are covered in fine, downy hairs. The herb is named for the uncanny effect it has on cats that are sensitive to it. Catnip contains the organic compound nepetalactone, which gives the herb its characteristic scent—a winsome blend of freshly mown grass and spearmint gum. When genetically sensitive cats inhale its scent, they will exhibit a state of euphoria and/or extreme playfulness—a reaction that lasts about ten minutes. In people, catnip acts as a mild nervine and sedative, calming the nerves and increasing drowsiness. Its leaves and flowering tops are used to make teas and tinctures. The young leaves can be pinched from the plant and eaten raw. Catnip has a gentle, soothing effect on the body and can be combined with chamomile (page 144) to make a relaxing tea. Considered to be a child-friendly herb, it is also an effective treatment for colds, upset stomachs, and the irritability and tension that may accompany these ailments.

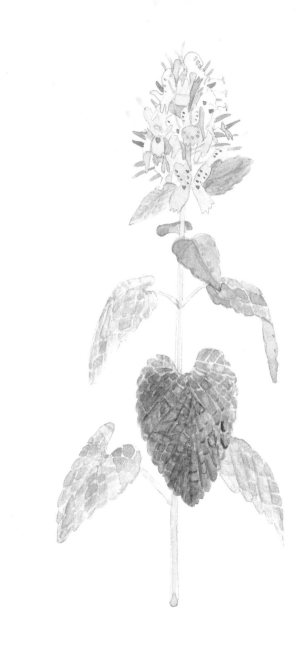

HAWTHORN & MIMOSA

{ **BOTANICAL NAMES:** *Crataegus laevigata*;
Albizia julibrissin
ORIGINS: Europe; Southwestern and
Eastern Asia }

When consumed in combination, hawthorn (bottom) and mimosa (top) form a powerful remedy for easing emotions such as sadness and grief. Hawthorn is a flowering shrub in the rose family with a long history of use as a gentle but highly effective medicine for strengthening the heart and circulatory system. Its leaves, flowers, and berries contain compounds that are thought to exert a normalizing effect on the heart, steadying the heartbeat and relieving palpitations. Extracts of hawthorn appear to dilate the arteries, reducing their constriction and helping to lower blood pressure. Hawthorn also acts as a nervine, reducing nervousness and tension, and a mild sedative, making it useful for stress-related sleep disorders and mild insomnia. Mimosa is a deciduous flowering tree, widely cultivated as an ornamental plant for its striking pink and white blossoms as well as its medicinal value. In traditional Chinese medicine, mimosa is referred to as *he huan pi*, which translates to "collective happiness bark." It has an uplifting effect on mood and appears to act as a mild antidepressant. When combined in a liquid extract or tincture, the two herbs work together to alleviate the heavy-hearted feeling many of us experience during difficult times, helping to relieve some of the physical effects of stress and improving mood.

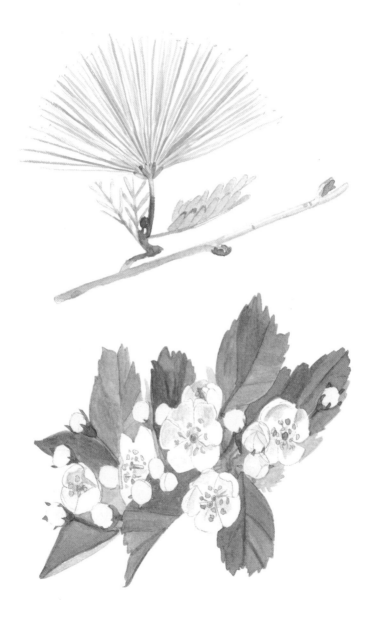

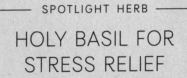

HOLY BASIL FOR STRESS RELIEF

As an herbal tonic for the nervous system, holy basil is cherished for its abilities to lift the spirits, improve mood, and promote relaxation. It is one of the most beloved plants in Indian folk medicine and Ayurveda, an ancient system of healing rooted in more than three thousand years of Indian culture. In Ayurvedic medicine, holy basil is known as a *rasayana*, a natural substance that promotes health and longevity. In India, it is widely known by the names *tulsi* and *tulasi*, which translate to "the incomparable one," reflecting the herb's cultural importance.

Though holy basil is native to India, it grows throughout tropical Asia, where it is commonly used in cooking, folk medicine, and spiritual practices, while herbal medicine practitioners around the world typically consume it in teas and tinctures. As a relative of the culinary herb sweet basil, holy basil shares its aromatic quality but has a unique scent and flavor of its own, with notes of clove, mint, and bubble gum. Its Latin name, *Ocimum tenuiflorum*, means "fragrant lipped slender flowers." The use of "holy" in its English common name derives from another previously used Latin name for the herb, *Ocimum sanctum*.

In contemporary herbal medicine, holy basil is highly valued for its ability to help alleviate stress. It's recognized both as a calming nervine that soothes the mind and as an adaptogenic herb with a normalizing effect on the body. Holy basil is thought to work in part by increasing circulation to the brain. This may help improve overall brain function, in turn reducing cloudy thinking and enhancing mental clarity.

Beyond its benefits to the nervous system, holy basil contains a bountiful bouquet of compounds with antibacterial, antiviral, antioxidant, and expectorant activity. These properties make the herb an ideal remedy whenever colds and coughs accompany stressful periods. It also contains a powerful combination of phytochemicals that are thought to give the herb its anti-inflammatory and stress-relieving properties.

LAVENDER

BOTANICAL NAME: *Lavandula angustifolia*
ORIGINS: Mediterranean Region and
North Africa

Lavender is an aromatic flowering herb that has been used in medicine and perfumery for more than twenty-five hundred years. It was valued among the ancient Greeks, Romans, and Egyptians for its soothing effects as well as its powerful disinfecting properties. Its name is thought to come from the Latin word *lavare* ("to wash"), as the herb was historically used in cleaning. Among the nearly forty species that belong to its genus, English lavender (shown here) is among the most commonly used in herbal medicine today. Though not native to England, the herb may have received this moniker thanks to the affections of Queen Elizabeth I, who is said to have adored the flavor and aroma of lavender in preserves, tea, and perfume. Lavender owes its enduring popularity to a unique combination of aromatic oils that have relaxing and uplifting effects. It is recommended for reducing irritability and nervousness, as well as the mild muscle tension and upset stomach that sometimes accompany stress, enabling better sleep, greater relaxation, and improved mood. It is commonly consumed in teas and tinctures alongside other herbs, such as passionflower (page 150) and chamomile (page 144) to treat stress-related insomnia.

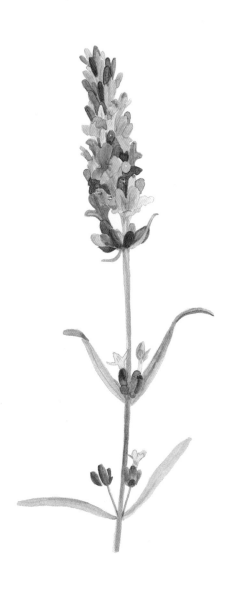

LEMON BALM

BOTANICAL NAME: *Melissa officinalis*
ORIGINS: Europe

Lemon balm is a well-known and beloved citrus-scented member of the mint family. Its leaves and flowering tops have been used for thousands of years across its native home of Europe, where its abilities to calm anxiety and lift spirits are legendary. The healthful benefits of lemon balm are noted in dozens of ancient texts and many early works on herbal medicine. The sixteenth-century English herbalist John Gerard wrote that "Bawme drunken in wine is good against the bitings of venomous beasts, comforts the heart, and driveth away all melancholy and sadness." Fragrant lemon balm leaves teem with aromatic oils and other compounds thought to contribute to its antianxiety and antiviral properties. The leaves are also beneficial for treating cold sores, which can be caused by stress and often in turn cause more stress. Lemon balm is a nervine that can help relieve a nervous stomach or the feeling of being overwhelmed, and it is an excellent remedy for treating seasonal affective disorder when paired with St. John's wort (page 78).

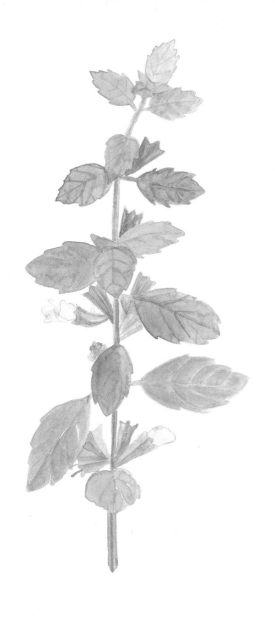

LINDEN

BOTANICAL NAME: *Tilia x europaea*
ORIGINS: Europe

Linden is an attractive, deciduous tree native to Europe, where it is commonly known as a "lime flower" or "lime tree," though it bears no relation to the sour citrus fruit of that name. Linden produces a thick coat of heart-shaped leaves and drooping clusters of blossoms. In the summer months, its flowers fill the surrounding air with the scents of honey and lemon peel. Linden belongs to a genus of about thirty trees, several of which have a long history of use in European folk medicine. They are now widely cultivated and thrive in temperate regions around the world. The flowers, bracts, and inner bark of two species of linden, *Tilia platyphyllos* and *Tilia cordata,* are commonly used to produce herbal teas and tinctures. The flowers contain aromatic oils, mucilage, and flavonoids—compounds with soothing nervine, antioxidant, and anti-inflammatory properties. Linden has a calming effect on mood and can be used as a very mild sedative for both adults and children. A tea or tincture of linden flowers helps to quell the irritability that often stems from ailments such as colds and coughs, headaches, and muscle tension.

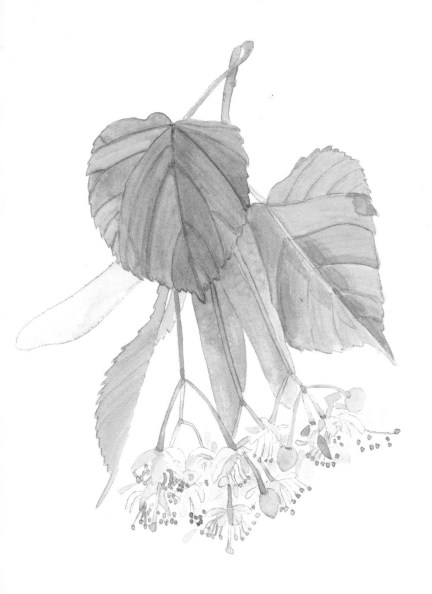

MILKY OAT SEED

{ **BOTANICAL NAME:** *Avena sativa*
ORIGINS: Mediterranean Region }

Milky oat seed comes from the seeds produced by the common oat plant, the same cereal grain grown to produce rolled oats and oatmeal. Oats are a member of the grass family; their relatives include wheat, barley, and rye. The immature seeds of oats are rich in vitamins, protein, and minerals. They are harvested and processed to make liquid extracts during a short window when oats are in their "milky stage," hence the common name of this well-known herb. In the nineteenth and twentieth centuries, American herbalists relied on milky oat seed for treating stress-related conditions and promoting healthy sleep patterns. Today milky oat seed is used for these general concerns, as well as specifically to calm anxious feelings and reduce irritability. It is considered both a nervine and a restorative herb that improves the general functioning of the nervous system, with a gentle, grounding effect that builds over time with use. Milky oat seed is an ideal long-term remedy for those with frayed nerves and a feeling of being burned out or mentally exhausted. It can be consumed on its own or combined with other nervine herbs.

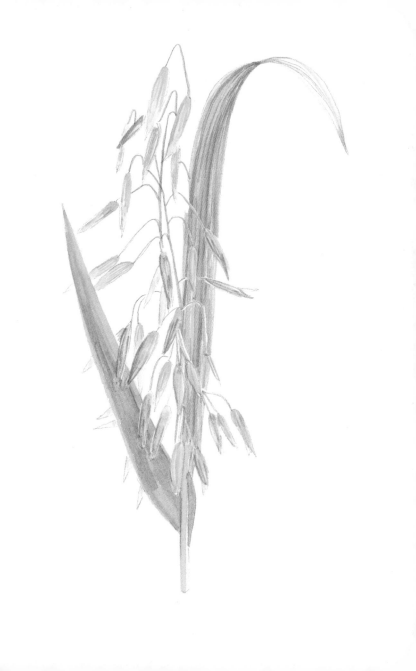

SKULLCAP

BOTANICAL NAME: *Scutellaria lateriflora*
ORIGINS: North America

Skullcap is a flowering herb traditionally used by Native Americans to treat a range of ailments related to the female menstrual cycle. European settlers readily adopted the use of skullcap but enlisted it primarily for nervous system conditions and for its antispasmodic properties. Today skullcap is recommended by herbalists to ease nervous tension and reduce anxiety. It contains several notable compounds including anti-inflammatory flavonoids and glutamine, an amino acid that plays a key role in the synthesis of proteins in the body. The majority of glutamine is stored in our muscles, where most of it is produced. When the body undergoes intense or prolonged physical or mentalstress, it may require greater levels of glutamine than it can produce on its own. The glutamine found in skullcap is considered to be partly responsible for its sedative and antianxiety effects. It is often recommended as a nervine to relieve stress-related exhaustion. Because of the delicacy of its phytochemical constituents, skullcap must be harvested and handled carefully to preserve its medicinal value. The flowering tops are typically gathered and processed into liquid extracts during the late spring and summer months, when the flowers are in peak bloom.

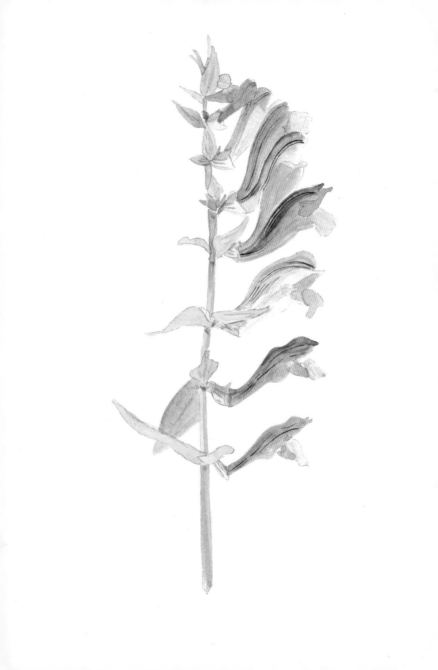

ST. JOHN'S WORT

BOTANICAL NAME: *Hypericum perforatum*
ORIGINS: Europe

St. John's wort has been used for thousands of years as a remedy for a wide range of ailments related to the nerves and central nervous system. The ancient Greek physician Hippocrates appears to have been the first to record the use of St. John's wort in the fifth century B.C.E. In the medieval European folk tradition, St. John's wort was revered as a protective herb and used to ward off illness. The herb may indeed offer such protection, as it has significant anti-inflammatory and pain-relieving properties. St. John's wort contains the compounds hypericin and hyperforin, both of which appear to exert neuroprotective effects. These two compounds, along with a group of nutrients called flavonoids, are considered the active elements responsible for the herb's uplifting effects. Hyperforin is an anti-inflammatory compound with antibacterial activity; hypericin has antiviral and antibacterial activity. Because of these properties, St. John's wort is widely used in conjunction with yarrow in wound healing (page 136) and often used to treat nerve pain. More broadly, St. John's wort is regarded as an herb that can be used to promote a sense of emotional well-being. Many herbalists recommend St. John's wort for mild anxiety, moodiness, and seasonal affective disorder.

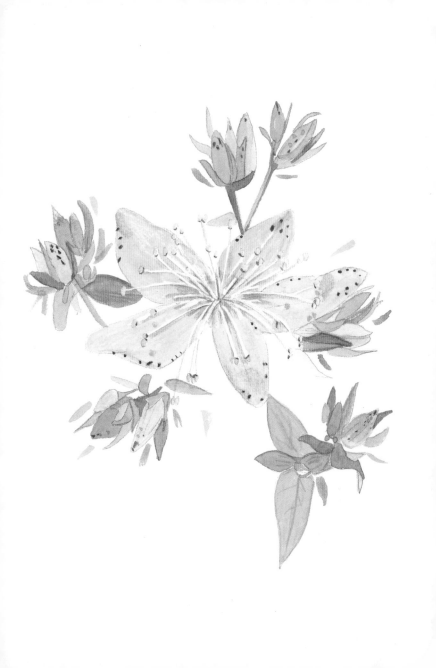

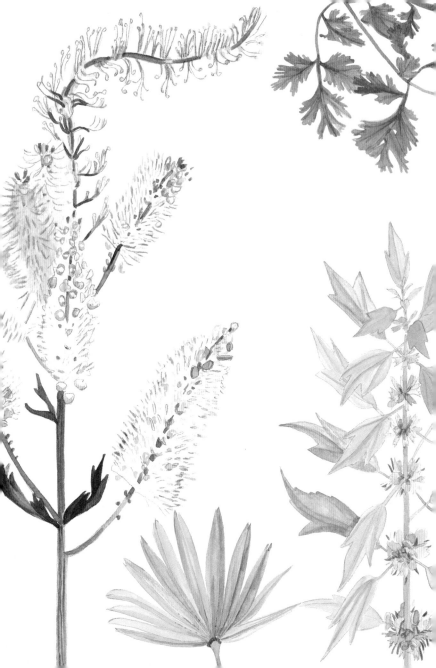

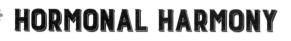

HORMONAL HARMONY

Hormones play major roles in our growth and development, and they regulate a multitude of bodily processes throughout our lives. The term *hormone* is based on the Greek word for "impetus," and it was coined in the early twentieth century to describe chemical messengers that appeared to coordinate activities in the body. Today we know that hormones regulate digestion, metabolism, reproduction, respiration, sleep, and stress. Acting as communicators between organs and tissues, they also influence movement and sensory perception. They are secreted by the endocrine system, a group of glands in the body, and have an enormous influence on our health, particularly as we age. At the same time, hormones often work quietly in the background, and their fluctuations tend to become routine. However, common ailments like hormonal acne or premenstrual tension can sometimes exaggerate regular cycles into longer slumps. Whether it's a monthly menstrual cycle or the declining testosterone levels that come with age, herbs offer trusted remedies that help the body adapt to these changes. This chapter highlights plants that can improve overall hormonal regulation and alleviate some of the symptoms of hormonal fluctuations. While not all of the herbs highlighted in this chapter influence hormones directly, all have beneficial effects on our sexual and reproductive health that may in turn promote and complement hormonal balance.

BLACK COHOSH

BOTANICAL NAME: *Actaea racemosa*
ORIGINS: North America

Black cohosh is a flowering woodland herb traditionally used by many eastern tribes of Native Americans, who consumed it as a remedy for lung and kidney ailments, pain, sore throat and cold symptoms, and muscle aches, spasms, and cramps. Since the mid-twentieth century, it has been popular in western Europe, where it's prescribed to help relieve menopausal symptoms, reduce premenstrual tension, and promote regular menstrual cycles. It's often recommended as a gentle, normalizing herb for both women and men during menopause and andropause, when hormone levels begin to fluctuate and decline. With impressively gnarled dark brown to black roots that are knobby with rugged and tough rhizomes, its form inspired the application of the Algonquin word *cohosh,* which means "rough." In contrast, its white flowers are fluffy and aromatic, exuding a slightly sweet fragrance reminiscent of cough syrup.

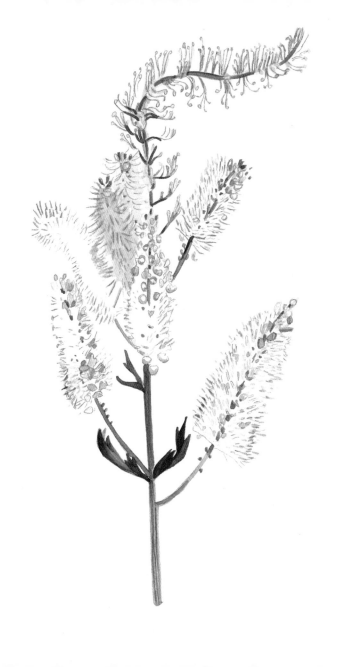

CHASTE TREE BERRY

{ **BOTANICAL NAME:** *Vitex agnus-castus*
ORIGINS: Southern Europe }

Chaste tree berry is widely cultivated for its beautiful foliage and butterfly-attracting flowers. In traditional herbal medicine, it is highly regarded for its ability to normalize the functioning of the male and female reproductive systems. The Greek physician Hippocrates recommended chaste tree berry for various gynecological conditions as early as the fourth century B.C.E. Since at least that time, it has been used to treat ailments related to female menstruation. Specifically, it can help promote regular and healthy menstrual cycles, balance key hormones such as progesterone and estrogen, and greatly reduce PMS symptoms such as hormonal acne, mood changes, fluid retention, and breast tenderness. Both the species name and common name of this herb arise from an unearned reputation. The terms *castus* and *chaste* refer to the long-disregarded medieval European notion that consuming the berries would promote chastity. Though it has acquired something of a reputation as a women's herb, chaste tree berry has also been shown to help men who are experiencing midlife andropause by promoting balanced hormone levels. It has a gentle, normalizing effect and works best when taken over time in capsules or tinctures.

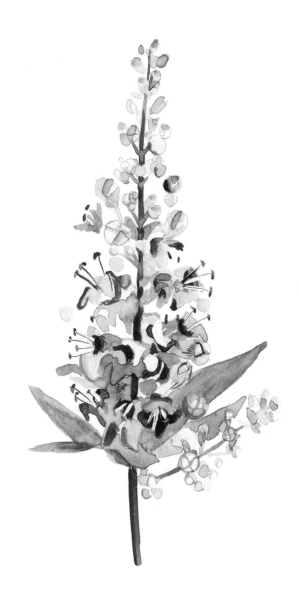

MOTHERWORT

BOTANICAL NAME: *Leonurus cardiaca*
ORIGINS: Central Asia and
Southeastern Europe

Motherwort is a flowering herb in the mint family that has spread throughout the world largely thanks to its use in herbal medicine. It takes its common name from its reputation as an herb for expectant mothers. In ancient Greece, pregnant women are said to have consumed motherwort to relieve uneasiness and reduce tension. Today motherwort is valued for its ability to promote healthy menstrual cycles. A mild emmenagogue—which is an herb that encourages blood flow in the pelvic area— it can gently prompt uterine contractions and help bring on delayed menses. Its species name, *cardiaca*, refers to its benefits beyond hormonal health as a treatment for ailments of the heart. As the seventeenth-century English herbalist Nicholas Culpeper wrote of motherwort, "There is no better herb to take melancholy vapors from the heart and make a merry, cheerful soul." In colonial America, Native Americans and Europeans used motherwort to brew a tea for calming nervous tension. Motherwort is often used today for reducing stress-related hypertension and treating heart palpitations. The aerial parts of the plant contain leonurine, a compound that appears to act as a mild vasodilator, which helps lower blood pressure. Motherwort also has nervine and antispasmodic properties, contributing to its ability to relieve stress and reduce tension.

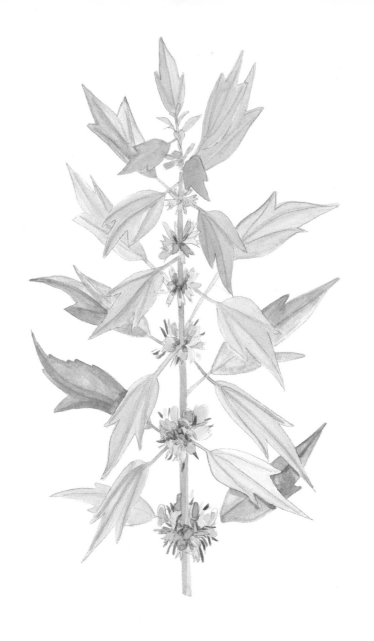

PARSLEY

BOTANICAL NAME: *Petroselinum crispum*
ORIGINS: Mediterranean Region

Parsley is so well known for its flavor and use as a culinary herb that its diverse healing benefits are often overlooked. Native to the Mediterranean, naturalized throughout Europe, and widely used in cooking from the Middle East to the Americas, it has many stamps on its passport and a history of use dating back more than two thousand years. It was much esteemed by the ancient Greeks, who not only consumed it but also used it as a garland to grace the necks of victorious athletes. Its anti-inflammatory properties make parsley an excellent aid for a range of urinary tract ailments in both men and women. It's also commonly used as an emmenagogue to gently stimulate menstruation and support healthy menstrual cycles. Parsley leaves contain two compounds in particular, apiol and myristicin, that are known to stimulate uterine contractions, which may help bring on delayed menses. As a versatile culinary herb, parsley may be eaten or brewed as a hot tea to further extract its beneficial compounds. Beyond its medicinal properties, parsley is also a rich source of antioxidants and nutrients, including significant amounts of calcium, magnesium, potassium, and vitamins A, C, and K.

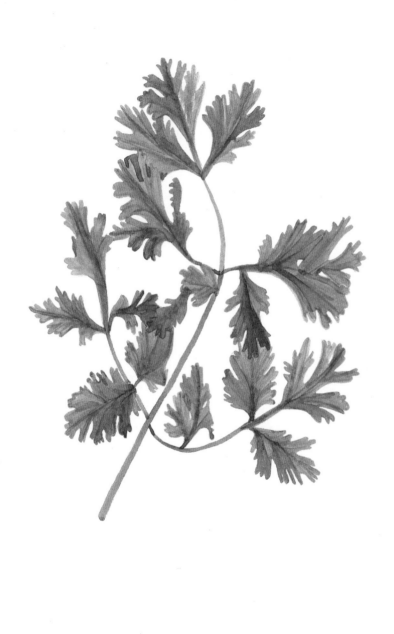

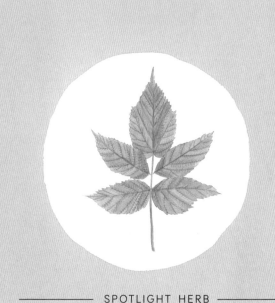

RASPBERRY LEAF FOR SEXUAL HEALTH

Raspberry leaf (*Rubus idaeus*), which is the leaf of the raspberry bush, is native to northern Eurasia. The bush is perhaps better known for its berries, which have been sought after for their deliciously sweet yet tart flavor since the time of the ancient Greeks. The Olympian gods were said to have discovered the berries growing on Mount Ida in Crete. This story is reflected in raspberry's botanical name, which means in Latin "bramble bush of Ida." The sixteenth-century English herbalist John Gerard was the first to describe the medicinal uses of the raspberry leaf, noting its astringent properties and use in treating stomach ailments.

Today raspberry leaf is considered to be an excellent tonic for both the male and female reproductive organs. It is especially valued for its ability to strengthen, relax, and tone the uterus, which in turn helps to reduce, and can ultimately eliminate, cramping related to menstruation. Raspberry leaf appears to relieve cramps partly by gently regulating uterine contractions, normalizing their frequency and intensity. Moreover, the vitamins and minerals abundant in raspberry leaves play a role in relaxing muscles, promoting healthy sleep patterns, and improving mood. Raspberry leaf also contains tannins with astringent properties that make it an ideal herb for alleviating stomach and bowel upsets. It also has anti-inflammatory properties and appears to help inhibit an enzyme in the body that is responsible for the formation of pain-causing compounds.

Raspberry leaf makes for a pleasant-tasting tea on its own or in combination with other herbs. It can be combined with red clover (page 92) and milky oat seed (page 92), or catnip (page 62) to make a relaxing and nutrient-rich drink that is enjoyable hot or cold. Because it's a gentle herb that can take several weeks to fully strengthen and tone the reproductive system, raspberry leaf generally works best when consumed regularly over time.

RED CLOVER & MILKY OAT SEED

BOTANICAL NAMES: *Trifolium pratense*;
Avena sativa
ORIGINS: Europe, Africa, and Western
Asia; Western Asia

Taken in combination, red clover (right) and milky oat seed (left) promote hormonal balance and support the nervous system, and are known to be particularly helpful to women during menopause, alleviating many of its symptoms and helping the body adapt to change. Red clover is rich in isoflavones, compounds known as phytoestrogens for their ability to produce estrogen-like effects, hence the herb's reputation as a treatment for menopausal symptoms. Milky oat seed (page 74) is considered a nervine that can be used to reduce the stress and irritability that can stem from hormonal changes. When combined in teas or tinctures, the two herbs may help improve mood and promote greater hormonal balance. Red clover has naturalized in many parts of the world and has played a role in agriculture and medicine for hundreds of years. It's widely cultivated by farmers as a cover crop and valued for its ability to fix nitrogen, an essential nutrient for plant growth, in the soil. As the state flower for Vermont, it symbolizes the state's agrarian heritage. In the folk medicine of many cultures, it is used to make a sweet-tasting tea that is valued for its anti-inflammatory, expectorant, and mildly sedative properties.

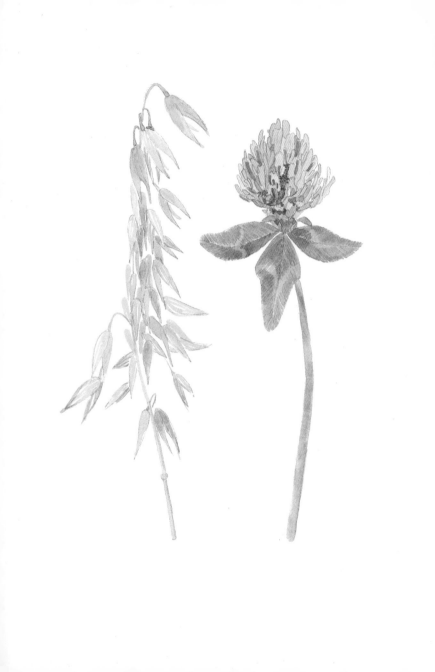

SAW PALMETTO

BOTANICAL NAME: *Serenoa repens*
ORIGINS: Southern United States

Saw palmetto is a small palm tree armed with saw-tooth spines that is native to the southeastern United States, where it sprawls in vast thickets across more than a million acres in the Florida Everglades. Thousands of tons of its berries are harvested annually for the herbal products industry. The berries resemble olives and ripen from light green to purplish black. It's thought that Native Americans consumed the berries as a food source for more than ten thousand years. The Seminoles relied on saw palmetto as both a staple and a medicinal plant, using it for urinary and digestive ailments. Well reputed as a men's herb, saw palmetto is now considered to be a premier herb for treating andrological conditions. Extracts from the berries strengthen the male reproductive system and work as an anti-inflammatory agent. Saw palmetto also has antiseptic properties that make it useful for treating urinary tract infections. It reduces urinary pain and discomfort and may help decrease the frequency of nighttime urination. Extracts also appear to improve the symptoms of an enlarged prostate gland. It's used by millions of men as a remedy for the discomfort caused by this common ailment.

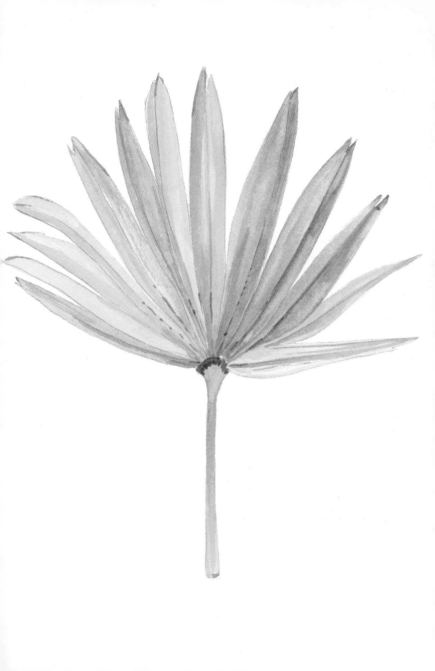

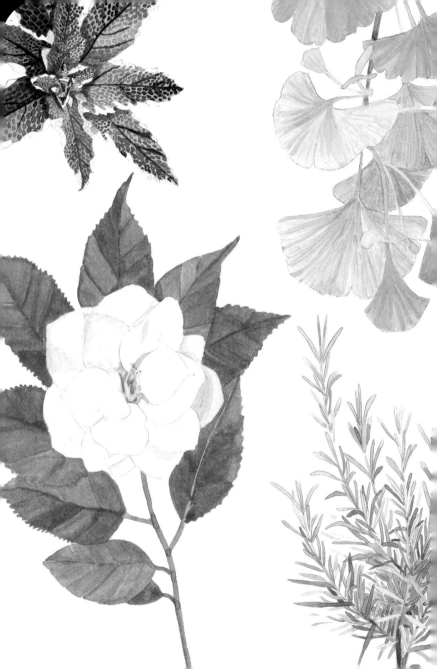

MENTAL CLARITY & FOCUS

The invigorating and mentally stimulating benefits of herbs have been appreciated since before recorded history. Indeed, as you'll read in the chapter ahead, our forebears left us with a rich global tradition of herbal medicine to support mental acuity at every stage of life. The challenge today is resisting the highly caffeinated, sugary drinks and calorie-packed snacks that, though they may give us spikes in energy and focus, often have a drop-off effect that only brings us back for more. Herbs are gently stimulating alternatives that don't tend to put us on a roller coaster of ups and downs. Powerhouses of nutrients, minerals, and phytochemicals, the herbs highlighted in this chapter deliver a balanced serving of energy and a delightful mélange of colors, flavors, and aromas that stimulate the senses and focus the mind.

GINKGO

BOTANICAL NAME: *Ginkgo biloba*
ORIGINS: China

Ginkgo trees are the oldest surviving tree species on earth, with fossil records dating back more than 270 million years. They are hardy trees, growing to up to 120 feet and thriving for 1,000 years or more. They are also perhaps the most fabulously clothed, featuring thin, smooth leaves that are fan-shaped and finely veined. In autumn, the leaves turn bright yellow and pattern the ground with brilliant color. They are dioecious, meaning that female and male flowers occur on separate trees. Female trees produce small yellow- to peach-colored fruits with a single seed that are attractive but have an unpleasant smell caused by the compound butyric acid. The seeds are valued in traditional Chinese medicine for their astringent properties. The contemporary use of ginkgo focuses on extracts made from the dried green leaves of the tree. One of the most widely used plant medicines in the world, ginkgo is believed to support circulation, memory, and mental clarity. Of the more than forty compounds identified in the leaves, two groups of nutrients are thought to be responsible for ginkgo's medicinal effects—antioxidant flavonoids and terpenoids, which dilate blood vessels.

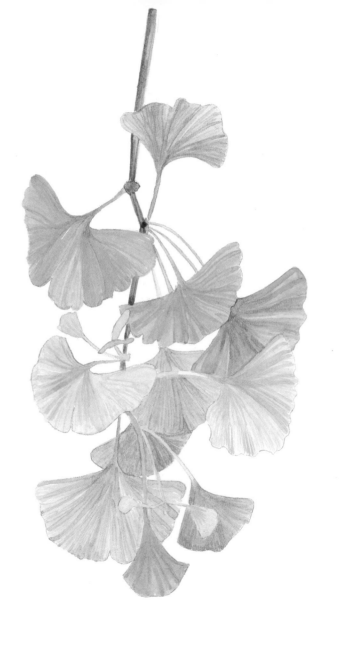

GREEN TEA, WHITE TEA

BOTANICAL NAME: *Camellia sinensis*
ORIGINS: Eastern Asia

Tea, made from leaves from the tea plant, has been consumed as a stimulating drink for thousands of years. The earliest known archeological evidence of tea consumption dates to the Han dynasty, more than twenty-one hundred years ago. Green tea and white tea are renowned for their energizing and health-enhancing properties. Green tea is made from mature leaves that have been allowed to oxidize and partially ferment before processing, while white tea is made from young leaves and buds that are minimally processed. An eight-ounce cup of white tea usually contains 20 to 40 mg of caffeine, whereas the same amount of green tea contains 50 to 70 mg. (The precise amount of caffeine in tea depends in part on the temperature of the water used and the length of time it's brewed.) Green and white teas contain antioxidants (with white tea known to contain a greater concentration of them) that have been linked to improved cardiovascular health, greater immunity, and enhanced central nervous system health. The combination of nourishing and stimulating compounds found in green and white teas makes them ideal for uplifting the mood and promoting mental clarity and focus.

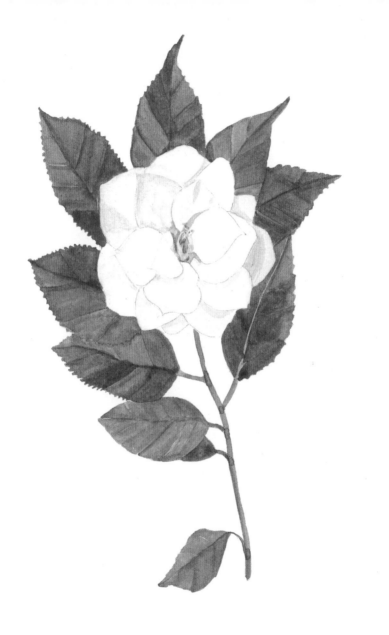

GOTU KOLA FOR NERVOUS SYSTEM HEALTH

Gotu kola has been used for thousands of years as a rejuvenating herbal tonic for the nervous system. Today it remains a common herb used to enhance mental performance. It is native to China, India, and Southeast Asia, where it is widely used in both food and folk medicine. The genus of its Latin name, *Centella asiatica*, is derived from the word for "hundred" and refers to its prolific growing habit. Essentially an aquatic plant, gotu kola spreads rapidly in wetlands, producing a thick mat of crescent-shaped leaves.

Gotu kola was first mentioned in the earliest Chinese pharmacopoeia, the *Shennong Bencaojing*, under the name *ji xue cao*, where it was recommended as a cooling, drying herb useful for relieving fevers and reducing inflammation. In the Ayurvedic tradition of India, gotu kola is considered an important herb for promoting longevity. It was listed in the *Sushruta Samhita*, an ancient Indian medical text written approximately two thousand years ago. It was considered useful for treating many types of physical and mental debility and for promoting convalescence. Traditionally, it has also been used along with other herbs such as withania (page 30) to counter age-related declines in mental function and cognition among the elderly. Gotu kola is obtainable as a fresh herb in its native range, and it is typically consumed in capsules and tinctures elsewhere.

Today gotu kola is regarded as a nootropic, a substance that improves mental function. It contains several compounds in its leaves that are thought to reduce mild anxiety and promote a state of relaxed focus. It may also improve mental clarity and memory retention. Beyond its benefits for mental performance, modern herbalists also view gotu kola as a premier herb for vascular health. It appears to strengthen the veins and support the regeneration of connective tissues, making it a potentially valuable herb for reducing the effects of aging.

ORANGE, APPLE & PINEAPPLE MINT

BOTANICAL NAMES: *Mentha citrata; Mentha suaveolens; Mentha suaveolens 'Variegata'*
ORIGINS: Mediterranean Region

Mint (*Mentha*) comes in more than two thousand named varieties. The best-known mints are spearmint and peppermint (page 56), but orange mint (top left), apple mint (top right), and pineapple mint (bottom) have much to recommend them, particularly from gardeners who favor them for their fantastic foliage and scents. Each of these mints is a hybrid developed partly through the selection of various desirable traits. They all retain the major health benefits of the better-known mints in that they soothe digestion, enhance concentration, and promote a state of relaxed focus. What's more, they add to the exceptional versatility of mint in cooking. Orange mint, redolent of citrusy fragrances ranging from grapefruit to lemon, can be used in salads, desserts, and drinks. Apple mint has a fresh, sweet aroma and is used in jellies, syrups, and drinks. Pineapple mint is a cultivar of apple mint, selected for its green-and-cream colored leaves and uncanny pineapple scent. Like other mints, it can be added to a variety of foods and drinks. Each of these varieties can be enjoyed as a pick-me-up at any time of the day. The cooling effects of mint are especially welcome on hot days when fatigue can start to set in, though they can be enjoyed any time of the year to clear away mental fog and enhance focus.

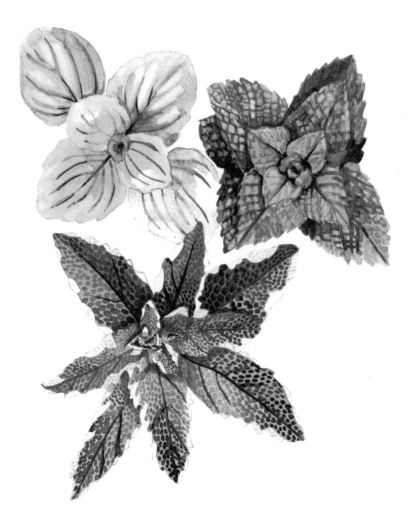

ROSEMARY

BOTANICAL NAME: *Rosmarinus officinalis*
ORIGINS: Mediterranean Region

Rosemary is perhaps best known as a culinary herb, but its fragrant needles also have a long history of use as a medicinal herb that can increase mental clarity, enhance concentration, and improve memory. This last benefit is claimed by no less than Shakespeare's Ophelia, who says, "There's rosemary, that's for remembrance; pray, love, remember," in *Hamlet*. Rosemary is thought to stimulate circulation and increase blood flow to the brain, resulting in a heightened state of focus. It also has significant antioxidant and anti-inflammatory properties. Its unique fragrance—enjoyed by many through aromatherapy—may help reduce stress levels and improve mood, in turn lowering the body's level of cortisol, a hormone associated with stress; it may also help relieve headaches, especially those brought on by stress.

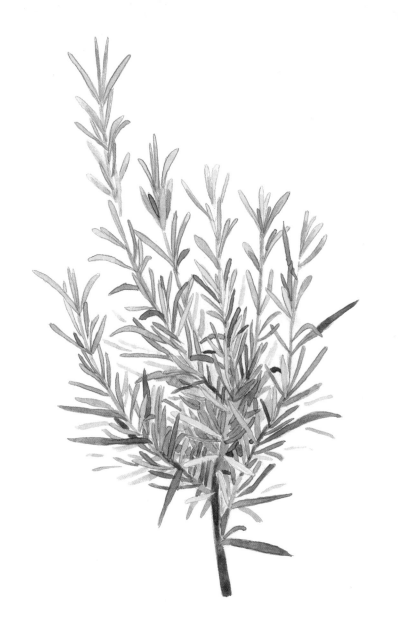

YERBA MATE

BOTANICAL NAME: *Ilex paraguariensis*
ORIGINS: South America

Yerba mate, a member of the holly family, contains caffeine and is widely consumed as a stimulating drink—prepared by steeping its dried leaves in hot water—throughout its native range of South America. There, mate is traditionally served in a hollow gourd and sipped using a *bombilla,* a metal straw that filters out the ground plant material. (In Spanish, *bombilla* also means "lightbulb," a fitting name for a tool used to consume such a mentally stimulating drink.) The amount of caffeine in an 8-ounce cup of yerba mate is estimated at 85 mg. Like other caffeinated drinks, yerba mate is consumed to boost concentration and increase energy, but it's also highly valued for being rich in nutrients. Yerba mate contains vitamins A, C, and E, as well as B-complex vitamins, and significant amounts of calcium, magnesium, iron, and potassium. Notably, a close cousin of yerba mate, known as *yaupon*, is thought to be the only native caffeine-containing plant in North America and offers similar benefits. The leaves of both herbs also contain impressive quantities of antioxidants and phytochemicals that help fight fatigue and enhance stamina.

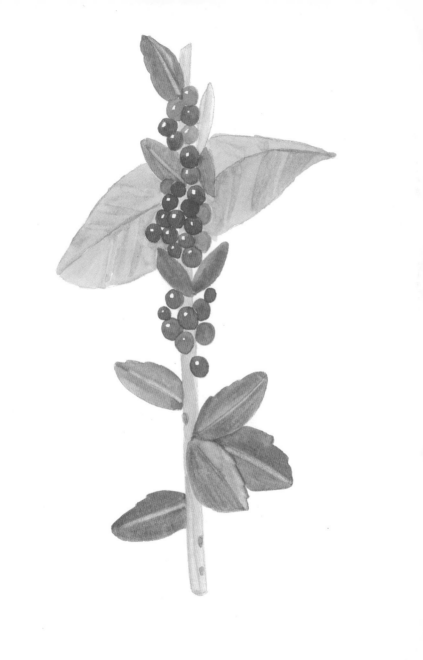

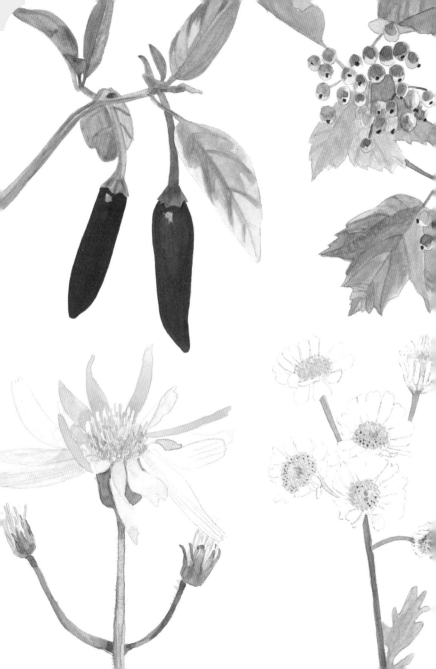

PAIN RELIEF

Throughout history, herbs have given us some of our most powerful and effective pain relievers. In his first-century pharmacopoeia, *De Materia Medica,* the Greek physician and botanist Dioscorides recommends dozens of herbs for hundreds of painful ailments. Indeed, many over-the-counter and prescription pain medicines in use today were first formulated from compounds discovered in plants many centuries ago. The herbs in this chapter, which include some of the oldest continuously used medicinal herbs in the world, are highly valued for their abilities to bring relief to life's everyday discomforts—the familiar aches, cramps, cricks, and pains—plus some types of chronic pain. Unlike conventional pain medicines that some-times mask the sensation of pain rather than address its underlying causes, herbs not only are known to relieve pain but may actually help decrease both the severity and frequency of pain over time. The herbs in this chapter are also among the easiest herbs to find. Some can even be found in the grocery store. Hint: check out the spice aisle when you're in the market for pain relief.

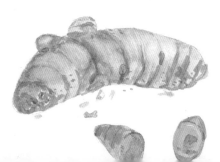

ARNICA

BOTANICAL NAME: *Arnica montana*
ORIGINS: Europe, Central Asia, and
North America

Arnica has been a trusted herb for pain relief for hundreds of years. In Europe, it plays a leading role in the traditional folk medicine of Germany, belonging to a group of herbs thought to have protective or healing properties called the *Zauberpflanzen*, which is German for "magic plants." Its origins as a healing herb in the United States date back to the latter half of the nineteenth century, when it was embraced by practitioners of eclectic medicine (a branch of medicine devoted to using botanical remedies), who used it as a treatment for external injuries and inflammation. Today arnica is widely used in topical salves and creams for relieving muscle pain, healing bruises, and soothing sprains. It exerts its anti-inflammatory effects on the skin, muscles, and skeletal system. Many types of injuries and ailments may be improved by using arnica, from backaches to painful ligaments and tendons. It's most effective when used immediately after injury but may also be used to improve chronic conditions such as joint pain. Notably, surgeons also sometimes recommend arnica to patients to aid in reducing bruising and swelling in postsurgery recovery.

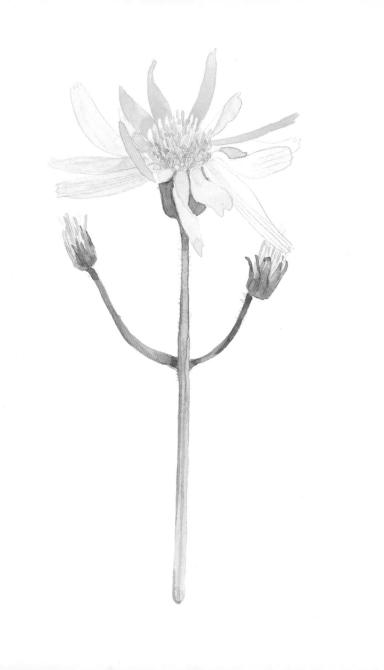

CAYENNE

BOTANICAL NAME: *Capsicum annuum*
ORIGINS: Tropical America

Cayenne is one of many cultivated varieties of capsicums, more commonly known as chiles or peppers. Archaeologists have unearthed evidence in Mexico that suggests humans have been consuming capsicums for at least nine thousand years. Cayenne is relished for the zesty kick it adds to foods and appreciated worldwide for its medicinal value. Its thin, vermilion flesh and small seeds contain constituents that give the cayenne pepper several healing benefits, including pain reduction, circulation boosts, and improved digestion. Capsaicin is the constituent that is responsible for both the intense heat of hot peppers and their pain-relieving properties. It is a rubefacient, a substance that warms and reddens the skin temporarily by dilating the capillaries and increasing circulation. Capsaicin appears to work by blocking the activity of a specific neurotransmitter called substance P, which relays pain information to the brain. Herbal salves made with cayenne are used to treat ailments in which increased blood flow and heat may be soothing, such as some types of headaches, sore muscles, and arthritis.

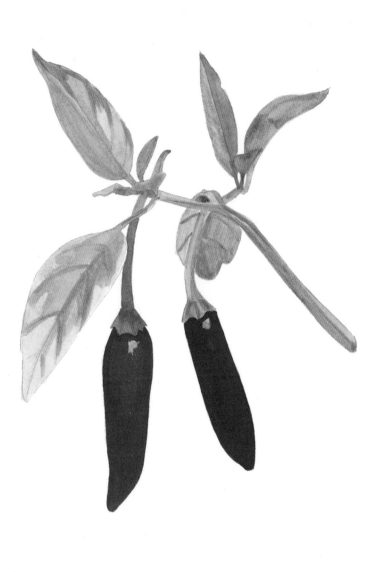

CRAMP BARK

BOTANICAL NAME: *Viburnum opulus*
ORIGINS: England and Scotland

Cramp bark is a shrub that is aptly and unforgettably named after its remarkable ability to alleviate cramps and pain. Cramp bark also has a close relative, known as black haw (*Viburnum prunifolium*), that contains many of the same constituents. The two herbs can be used interchangeably for most remedies as both have significant antispasmodic and pain-relieving properties. Cramp bark produces lightly fragrant bouquets of white flowers and drooping clusters of bright red berries. Historically, Native Americans, including the Iroquois and the Ojibwa, consumed the berries as a food and as a medicine to treat blood conditions. The inner bark of the shrub was harvested and boiled to make a medicine for alleviating pain. Today cramp bark is used as a remedy for relieving muscle spasms, low back pain, and abdominal cramps, as well as uterine cramps related to the menstrual cycle. It may also be helpful for treating tension headaches and some types of migraines. Cramp bark contains coumarins, scopoletin, and tannins—compounds with blood-thinning, anti-inflammatory, and astringent properties. The amount and combination of these compounds found in cramp bark is thought to help gently normalize blood pressure and relax muscle tissues.

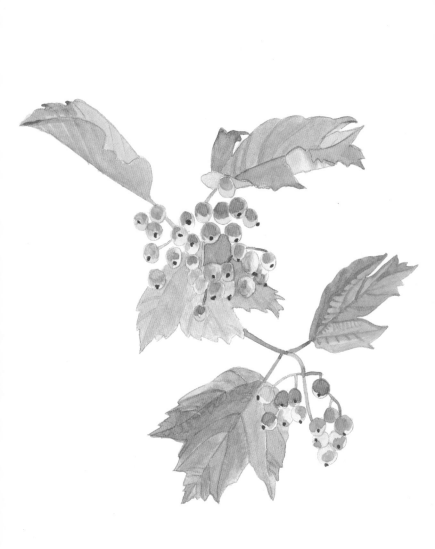

FEVERFEW

BOTANICAL NAME: *Tanacetum parthenium*
ORIGINS: Europe

Feverfew is a flowering herb with an unusually bitter scent that stems from its unique phytochemistry. Its common name comes from the Latin word *febrifugia* for "fever reducer." For more than two thousand years, feverfew has been used to treat a wide array of ailments, including fevers, headaches, nausea, tinnitus, arthritis, stomachaches, and toothaches. The Greek physician and botanist Dioscorides recommended feverfew for these maladies as well as for various gynecological conditions in his first-century text *De Materia Medica*. Today feverfew is highly regarded as a remedy used to reduce the frequency and severity of migraines. Its leaves and flowers contain parthenolide, a compound that appears to act as both an antispasmodic (which reduces muscle spasms) and a vasodilator (which lowers blood pressure). Each of these properties is thought to contribute to its pain-relieving effects. Feverfew may be consumed as a liquid extract or tincture, though the consumption of one of its fresh leaves a day is more common as a traditional remedy for preventing migraines. Fortunately, growing feverfew is nearly effortless, making it easy to have close at hand for such daily use.

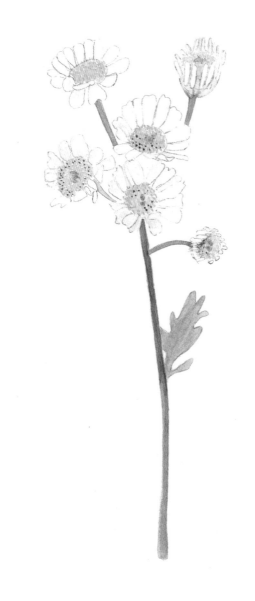

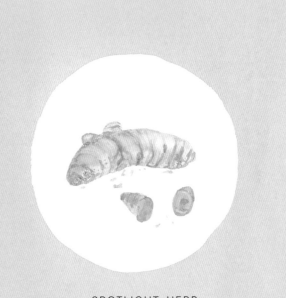

TURMERIC FOR INFLAMMATION

Turmeric (*Curcuma longa*) root has been used as a culinary spice, an additive to cosmetics, and a medicine for thousands of years across tropical Asia. It is a common spice used in Indian cuisine and gives curry powder its distinctive orange color. In traditional Chinese and Indian medicine, turmeric is valued as an herbal tonic for its ability to normalize systems in the body. In the folk traditions of both countries, it was used for promoting a healthy digestive system as well as for pain relief and skin care.

Turmeric belongs to the same family as ginger (page 40) and shares its anti-inflammatory and antimicrobial properties. In the area of pain relief, however, turmeric has few rivals among other plants or prescriptions. It works in part by reducing the levels of inflammatory chemicals in the body. Much like cayenne (page 114), it decreases the amount of substance P—a neuropeptide responsible for sending pain signals to the brain—in the nerve endings.

Beyond its properties as a pain reliever, turmeric aids in mental clarity and digestive health. The powerful antioxidant compound known as curcumin is found in large amounts in turmeric. It's also the pigment that gives turmeric roots their brilliant orange hue. Curcumin may act as a neuroprotective agent, reducing the buildup of protein-based plaques in the brain that are linked to Alzheimer's disease. Curcumin crosses the blood–brain barrier and binds to these plaques, helping clear them from the brain. Also known to have a normalizing effect on digestion, turmeric enhances the function of the liver and gallbladder and promotes healthy levels of intestinal flora. It also generally reduces irritation in the bowel and may protect against inflammatory bowel conditions. It's widely used as a remedy for alleviating upset stomach, cramps, and various liver and digestive ailments.

WHITE WILLOW BARK

BOTANICAL NAME: *Salix alba*
ORIGINS: Asia and Europe

White willow bark holds an important place in both folk medicine and modern medicine. Its pain-relieving effects were recognized by the ancient Greek physician Hippocrates, who is believed to have prescribed it for headaches. The bark contains salicin, an anti-inflammatory compound that takes its name from white willow's Latin genus, *Salix*. Notably, white willow bark is the original source of the world's best-known pain reliever, aspirin. In 1763, Englishman Edward Stone experimented with powdered white willow bark, successfully using it to treat pain and fever. But it was not until decades later that scientists extracted the active constituent of the bark, salicin, and isolated the crystalline compound salicylic acid. Their work ultimately led to the development of aspirin. However, chemical isolation isn't necessary to enjoy the benefits of white willow bark—our bodies can metabolize salicin and break it down into salicylic acid. White willow bark extract is widely available in tinctures and capsules, and the bark may also be made into a decoction or tea. It's considered to be gentle on the stomach and is often likened to taking a dose of "baby aspirin." It tends to work more slowly than pharmaceutical pain relievers but may also have longer-lasting effects.

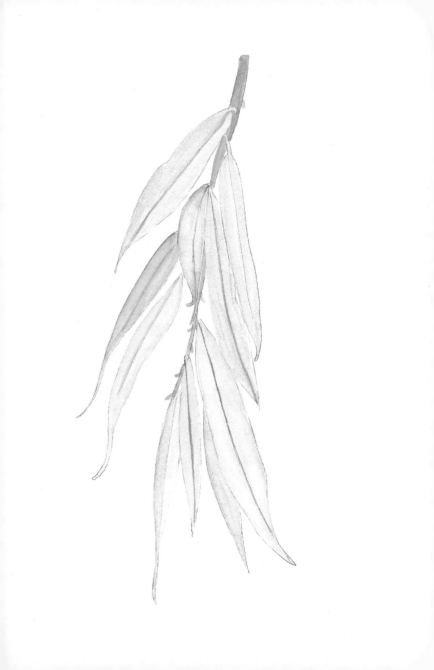

WOOD BETONY

BOTANICAL NAME: *Stachys officinalis*
ORIGINS: Europe

Wood betony is a perennial flowering herb native to the grasslands of Europe and naturalized in North America. It produces spikes of purplish flowers and its long, lance-shaped leaves—which contain glands that exude an aromatic oil—are covered in a prickly fur of fine hairs. Its history of use in medicine dates to the ancient Greeks and Romans, and in the fourth century, *De Herba Vettonica*, a lengthy tract describing more than forty ailments that could be treated by wood betony, was published. Wood betony was among the most highly valued plants in European folk medicine during the fifteenth century, when it was grown in monasteries and physic gardens, which were gardens that served as living pharmacies before pharmaceutical drugs were widely available. All parts of the herb were used to prepare remedies, such as teas and decoctions, for headaches, nervous tension, and muscle pain. Today wood betony is widely regarded as a nervine. It contains compounds with significant anti-inflammatory and antioxidant properties, including caffeic acid, chlorogenic acid, and rosmarinic acid, which collectively appear to exert a gently relaxing effect on the body.

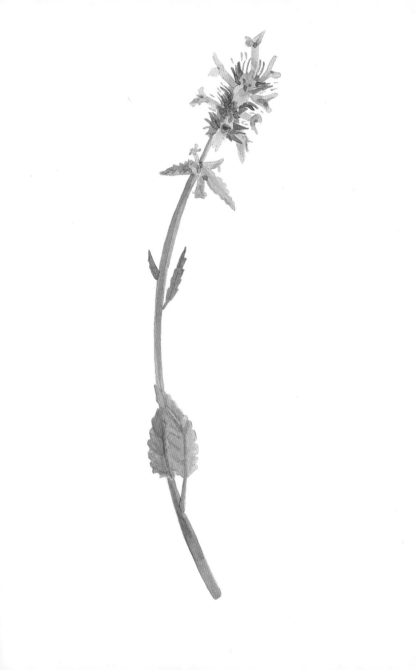

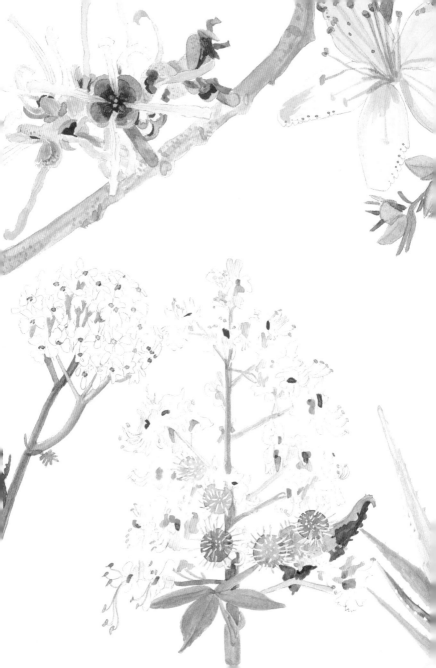

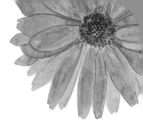

SKIN CARE

Our skin, which does the often thankless job of protecting us through thick and thin, plays a huge role in our everyday comfort and well-being, but we don't often give it the loving care it deserves. Minor skin ailments like cuts, bruises, chafing, acne, and other blemishes afflict us all at some point. Fortunately, the body has an impressive ability to heal itself, continuously repairing and replacing the skin to keep us well protected from childhood through old age. The herbs in this chapter help expedite and improve this natural process, making the sometimes unpleasant but vital healing that accompanies it easier to manage. They also help relieve inflammation and improve the appearance of skin. Without a doubt, the skin is our first layer of defense, but it can also be our first layer of delight. Having healthy skin feels good physically, and it can have a positive effect on the way we feel emotionally. Healing herbs are essential allies in keeping that most conspicuous part of our bodies healthy.

ALOE VERA

BOTANICAL NAME: *Aloe vera*
ORIGINS: Canary Islands, North Africa,
and Mediterranean Region

Aloe vera has been used in herbal medicine for thousands of years. The plant is mentioned in ancient Egyptian papyri dating from the sixteenth century B.C.E. It also appears in *De Materia Medica*, the herbal encyclopedia written by the Greek physician and botanist Dioscorides, where it is noted for its use in healing wounds and soothing rough skin. Because aloe vera has been cultivated for so long, a single point of geographic origin for the species remains somewhat unclear. Today aloe is grown in diverse regions around the world. It's also one of the easiest plants to grow indoors, which has made it a favorite of apartment dwellers everywhere. Aloe is perhaps the world's best-known succulent, a class of plants that evolved to retain water by storing it in their thick, fleshy leaves, stems, and roots. This has made aloe valuable as both a food and a medicine to people living in arid regions. Aloe helps to hydrate and lubricate the skin, reducing dryness and irritation. Its leaves contain a mucilaginous gel that is used to coat the skin. Aloe is safe to use on all parts of the body, provides relief to sunburned skin, and helps heal minor abrasions. It can be applied multiple times a day to enhance its soothing effects.

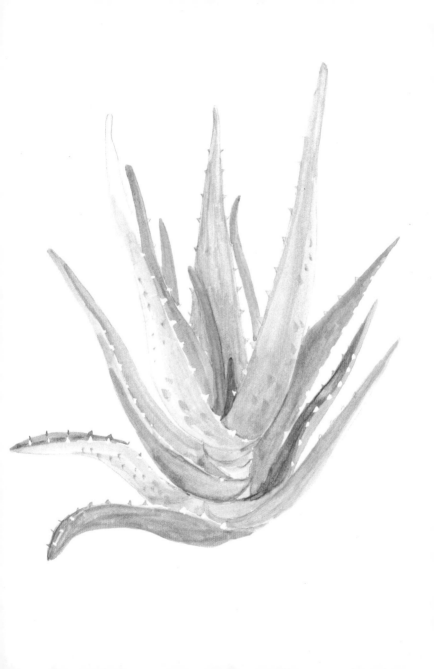

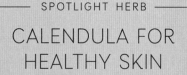

CALENDULA FOR HEALTHY SKIN

Calendula (*Calendula officinalis*) is one of the greatest first-aid remedies in herbal medicine and has a long history of use as an edible, cosmetic, ornamental, and decorative herb. The plant produces bright yellow-orange flowers and blooms throughout its growing season. It is native to the Mediterranean region, but thanks to its abundant and attractive growth, calendula has found a welcome home in gardens across the United States and Europe, where it has been cultivated since at least the twelfth century. In medieval

England, calendula flowers were traditionally used to treat toothaches, fevers, and digestive ailments.

Today calendula is widely regarded as an all-purpose tonic for promoting healthy skin. It's commonly used to alleviate a wide variety of skin conditions, including acne, burns, dry skin, minor cuts, insect bites, and athlete's foot. Calendula is a remarkably safe and gentle herb to use with children and can be helpful for treating many childhood and infantile ailments, such as ear infections and diaper rash. As a first-aid medicine, it is a highly valued vulnerary, or herb used for healing wounds. It also has anti-inflammatory properties that make it ideal for treating many forms of dermatitis, such as dandruff, eczema, and rashes.

Calendula flowers contain a number of potent compounds, including saponins and triterpenoids, phytochemicals with significant anti-inflammatory, antifungal, and antimicrobial qualities. The flowers also have astringent and styptic properties, which contribute to calendula's ability to sanitize and close wounds. This appears to work partly by promoting blood flow and tissue growth at the wound site. The flowers' astringent properties help firm the skin as it heals. While it's an excellent first-aid remedy for recent cuts and wounds, it also works well on older wounds that are slow to heal. It can be applied directly to clean wounds, whether closed or open. Applied to an open wound, calendula's styptic action staunches bleeding. Calendula is also commonly available in herbal oils, salves, and creams.

HORSE CHESTNUT

BOTANICAL NAME: *Aesculus hippocastanum*
ORIGINS: Southeastern Europe

Horse chestnut is a deciduous tree native to southeastern Europe and is cultivated around the world for its medicinal value. Though the tree bears the name "chestnut," it is not related to the chestnut that we often associate with winter holidays. You'll never roast a horse chestnut and eat it because, while horse chestnuts have medicinal value, they aren't actually edible. Only processed extracts from the seeds are used in herbal medicine today. In European folk tradition, horse chestnut was used to reduce swelling and help relieve injuries like sprains and bruises. Today extracts from horse chestnut seeds are used to heal ailments that affect the skin. The key active compound in the seeds is aescin, which inhibits the release of enzymes that degrade collagen, a protein found in our bones, skin, muscles, and all of our connective tissues. The compound is thought to help strengthen not only our skin but also our veins, improving their overall elasticity and enhancing the function of the circulatory system.

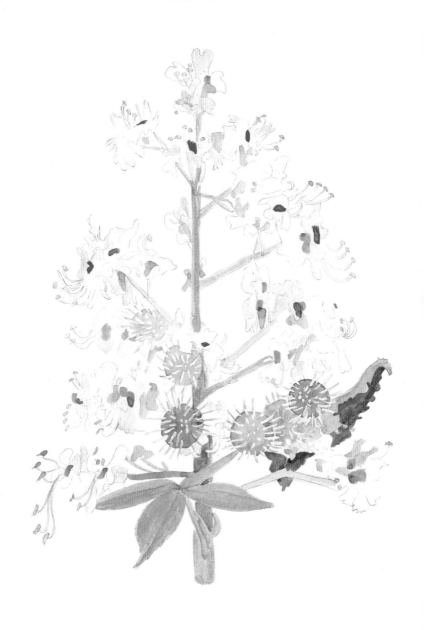

PLANTAIN

BOTANICAL NAME: *Plantago major*
ORIGINS: Europe and Central Asia

Referring not to the banana-like tropical tree by the same name but to the common wild herb, plantain is a noble weed indeed. Its leaves have long been used across Europe and North America as a traditional folk remedy for cleaning and healing wounds. A highly adaptable, wind-pollinated herb, plantain can be found in abundance on almost every continent. An equally common species is *Plantago lanceolata*. Plantain is a nutritious, vitamin- and mineral-rich edible plant with multiple uses, but it is perhaps best known as a "drawing agent," used to remove dirt and debris from wounds and draw out venom from the sites of stings and bites. Consider the herb's growing habits, and this unusual property may make a bit more sense. Botanists and herbalists alike have noted that plantain thrives in hard, compacted earth and exhibits a strong ability to draw nutrients from the soil with its hardy taproot. Plantain also has anti-inflammatory and pain-relieving properties, making it an ideal ingredient in salves and poultices used for wound care. Thanks to its distribution and usefulness, it's now one of the most widely used medicinal plants in the world.

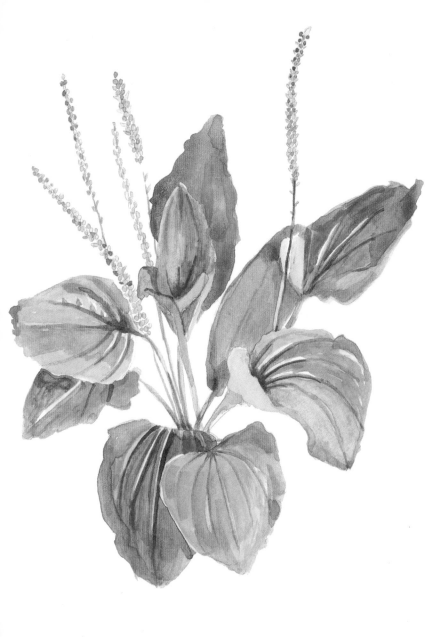

ST. JOHN'S WORT & YARROW

BOTANICAL NAMES: *Hypericum perforatum*; *Achillea millefolium*
ORIGINS: Europe; Asia and Europe

St. John's wort (left) and yarrow (right) have long histories as remedies for injuries to the skin. Used in combination, as in a salve or herbal oil applied to the skin, the herbs work together to speed healing of minor wounds. St. John's wort received its name from its association with Saint John the Baptist. It is said to bloom around the time of his birthday in late June. Its flowers emit a blood-red oil when bruised, which captured the imaginations of medieval Europeans and contributed to its legend. Its flowers have anti-inflammatory properties and can be applied to the skin to help heal bruises and burns. Yarrow has styptic, analgesic, and antiseptic properties, meaning that it halts bleeding, reduces pain, and helps prevent infection. The flowering tops and young leaves of the plant are typically used in herbal medicine. Famed botanist Carl Linnaeus gave yarrow its botanical name in 1753. He used *Achillea* to refer to Achilles, the mythological Greek hero of the Trojan War, who is reputed to have treated his soldiers' arrow wounds with yarrow. The word *millefolium* means "thousand leaves" and refers to the fine, lacy leaflets of the herb, which can be crushed and used to staunch wounds.

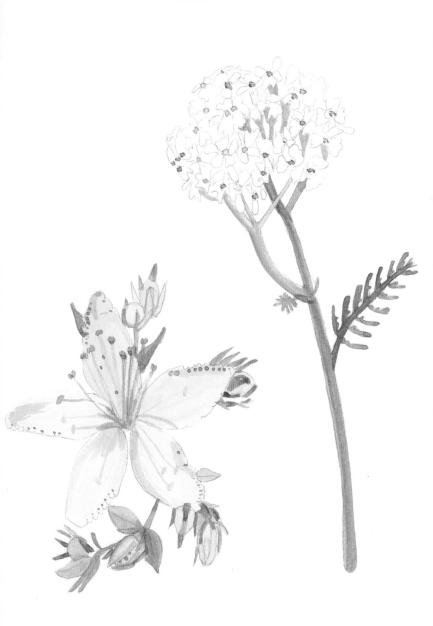

WITCH HAZEL

BOTANICAL NAME: *Hamamelis virginiana*
ORIGINS: Eastern North America

Witch hazel is a woodland shrub that produces a flourish of curly, crinkly yellow flowers in autumn. Native Americans used witch hazel leaves and bark for hundreds of years to relieve pain, soothe the skin, and treat cold symptoms such as fever and sore throat. Its name refers not to any sort of witchcraft, but derives from the old English *wych*, a word used to describe trees with pliable branches. As its leaves and branches resembled European hazel trees, English settlers to North America simply applied the same common name to the species. Witch hazel has mild astringent, anti-inflammatory, and antiseptic properties that make it ideal for treating a wide variety of skin conditions. It contains tannins, which are water-soluble compounds that impart astringency and bitterness to plants. Witch hazel has been used in commercial health products since the 1800s and remains commonly available in drugstores today, although the concentration of its extracts used in different products varies considerably. Some preparations are alcohol based and may be overdrying to the skin, while others are water based and are generally milder. As a natural astringent, witch hazel can be used to remove excess oil from the skin and help shrink pores, which may help treat and prevent blemishes.

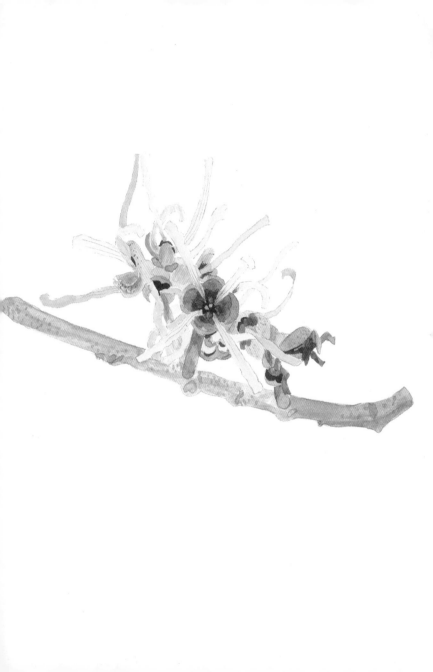

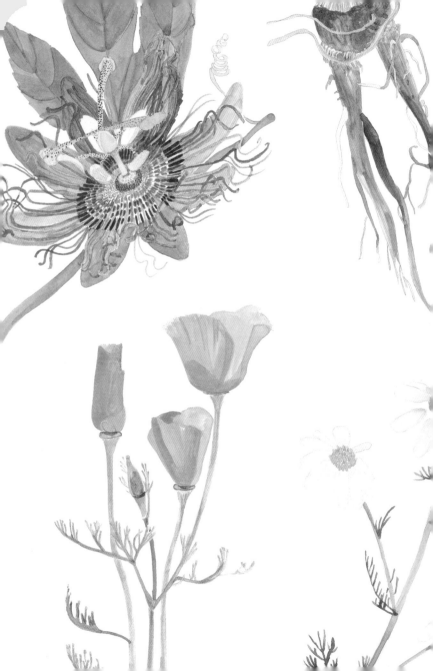

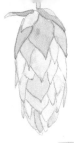

IMPROVED SLEEP

For thousands of years, we have looked to herbs for sleep aids. As early as the first century, the Greek physician and botanist Dioscorides wrote of the sleep-inducing effects of herbs. An activity that we spend an average of nearly one-third of our lives doing, sleep is crucial for brain health, muscle repair, hormonal balance, and immunity. Most of us know this instinctively because we've experienced the physical exhaustion and mental fog that descends when we don't get enough of it. On the other hand, little in life comes close to the blissful feeling of a good night's rest. The herbs in this chapter offer safe, natural remedies for improving the quality of your sleep and fine-tuning that vital one-third of your life, helping to alleviate problems with falling asleep, treat mild insomnia, and address sleep-maintenance problems such as waking up in the middle of the night. Commonly enjoyed in soothing teas or tinctures, herbal sleep aids can help relieve tension and restlessness, allowing you to drift off to sleep and wake up feeling rejuvenated the next day.

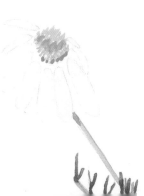

CALIFORNIA POPPY

{ **BOTANICAL NAME:** *Eschscholzia californica* }
ORIGINS: North America

California poppy, the state flower of California, is an edible wild plant whose botanical name memorializes Johann Eschscholtz, an Estonian physician who accompanied a Russian sailing expedition to California in the early nineteenth century. He and the crew collected samples of the flowers that covered the hillsides and gave the landscape a magnificent golden glow. Early Spanish explorers called it *copa de oro*, or "cup of gold," which is another of its common names. Native Americans in the region traditionally used the aerial parts of the plant for sleeplessness, nervousness, headaches, and to soothe stomach upsets. The stem and leaves of the plant were also cooked and eaten as a vegetable or potherb. Today the roots, leaves, and flowers of the plant are harvested and typically processed to produce liquid extracts while they're still fresh. The dried herb can also be used for making tea. Both of these preparations are noted for their sedative and relaxing effects and can be used to help promote a longer, more restful night's sleep.

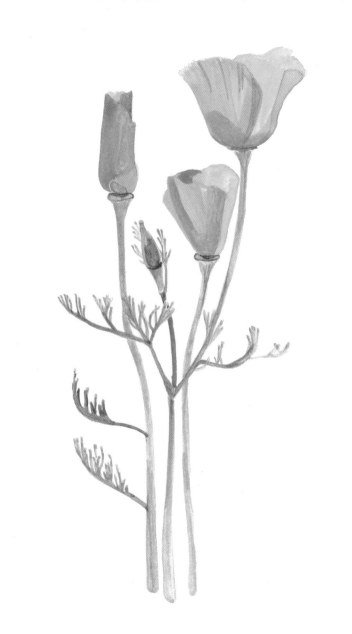

GERMAN CHAMOMILE FOR RESTFUL SLEEP

German chamomile has been used for thousands of years across its native regions of Europe and North Africa. The word *chamomile* comes from the Greek term *chamaimēlon*, which loosely translates to "apple on the ground" and evokes the sweet, apple-like scent of the plant. German chamomile (*Matricaria recutita*), which is shown above, is prized in herbal medicine because of its high concentration of healing compounds. A similar herb known as Roman chamomile (*Chamaemelum nobile*) shares its properties and has been used historically to treat the same range of ailments. While both herbs are common, German chamomile is more widely cultivated around the world and is often referred to simply as *chamomile*.

The ancient Greeks, Romans, and Egyptians revered chamomile and used its flowers and leaves medicinally for a wide range of ailments such as colds and coughs, wounds, digestive complaints, and gynecological problems. Chamomile's reputation as a tonic, cure-all herb is well deserved as it continues to be used to improve these conditions and many others. Today chamomile is cherished for its abilities to calm tension, ease anxiety, and induce a restful sleep. It is also widely used for its ability to soothe digestive ailments, which can make it difficult to fall asleep easily, and to provide relief for indigestion, flatulence, and nausea. Chamomile flowers also contain anti-inflammatory and antispasmodic compounds that relieve pain, cramps, and soreness, soothing the body and creating a more restful state.

More than 120 chemical constituents have been identified in chamomile. Notably, it contains chamazulene, an aromatic compound responsible for the brilliant blue oil that chamomile yields when distilled. This compound has anti-inflammatory action and is thought to contribute to the herb's skin-healing abilities. The sedative effects of chamomile are thought to come from its abundance of a compound called apigenin that appears to act as a relaxant on the central nervous system.

HOPS

BOTANICAL NAME: *Humulus lupulus*
ORIGINS: Europe, Southwest Asia,
and North America

Hops is the common name of an aromatic plant in the Cannabaceae family whose most notable relative is *Cannabis sativa*, or marijuana. While the resemblance doesn't go too far (hops won't get you high), the two plants have a few things in common. They both produce female and male flowers on the same plant and have a long history of cultivation and use as traditional remedies for sleeplessness and pain management. The word *hops* refers to the female flowers or cones of the herb, which are used in brewing beer and as a traditional remedy for nervousness and insomnia. Today hops are commonly used to make herbal teas and tinctures. A varied bouquet of aromatic and bitter compounds is thought to be responsible for these sedative and nervine properties. In hops, we also find linalool, myrcenol, pinene, and humulene. These same compounds are the building blocks of fragrance and flavor in many plants, from cannabis to oregano. The soothing scents and relaxing properties of hops have been enjoyed for hundreds of years, sometimes inadvertently. Early hops growers in Europe noticed that workers harvesting hops tended to be a drowsy bunch and often fell asleep on the job, cuing them into the potent sedative powers of the herb.

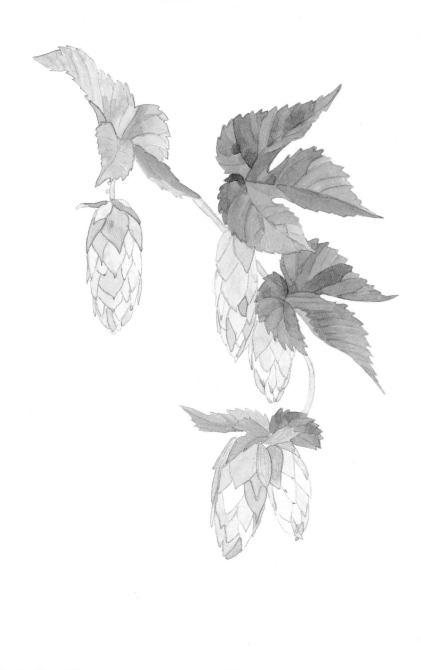

KAVA

BOTANICAL NAME: *Piper methysticum*
ORIGINS: Polynesia

Kava is an excellent herbal remedy for sleeplessness and insomnia noted for its ability to alleviate nervous tension and induce a deep, dreamless sleep. It is a Polynesian plant whose roots have been used for hundreds of years to brew a traditional drink consumed across the Pacific Islands. The drink is used both ceremonially and recreationally on many islands today and has become popular in the United States and Europe, where it is also commonly available in capsules and tinctures. Kava contains compounds called kavalactones that are thought to be responsible for many of its medicinal effects. Kavalactones exert a calming influence on the central nervous system and have shown pain-relieving, anti-anxiety, and sedative effects. Thanks to these properties, kava acts as a mild muscle relaxant and may help reduce the amount of time it takes to fall asleep. The amount of kava largely helps determine its effects: less concentrated amounts may be used for relaxation, while more concentrated amounts help induce sleep. Unless you live in the Pacific Islands, kava is best purchased from an herbal medicine company that fairly and sustainably harvests it.

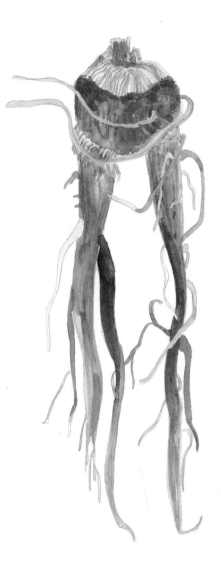

PASSIONFLOWER

{ **BOTANICAL NAME:** *Passiflora incarnata*
ORIGINS: North, Central, and South America }

Indigenous people throughout the Americas have cultivated passionflower for hundreds of years. William Strachey, the first secretary of the Jamestown colony, described the pleasant taste of passionflower fruit in his 1612 account and observed that "in every field where the indigenous people plant their Corne be Cart-loades of them." Native Americans used passionflower leaves, roots, and fruit for food, drink, and medicine. Despite any associations with its name, passionflower does not act as an aphrodisiac. Its name was given by early Christian missionaries to the Americas who believed the flower symbolized the Passion of Christ. Passionflower's stems, leaves, and flowers contain flavonoids, antioxidants, and alkaloids and are the parts typically used in herbal medicine. Passionflower appears to promote relaxation by acting on the central nervous system, where it increases the level of the brain's major inhibitory neurotransmitter, gamma-amino butyric acid, or GABA. This chemical works to inhibit nerve impulses and the activity of some brain cells, helping one feel calm and relaxed. Passionflower is especially effective for calming the nerves and quieting the mind before bedtime. It's also a great remedy for people who have trouble winding down as it reduces excitability. People with high-energy or demanding jobs may benefit from using passionflower for relaxation and improved sleep.

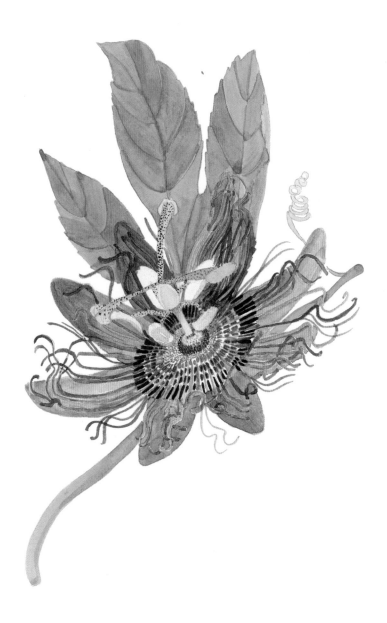

GLOSSARY OF HERBAL PROPERTIES

Medicinal herbs often have multiple properties that benefit the body. Here is a list of the most common properties you'll encounter during your exploration of herbal medicine, many of which appear in the pages of this book.

Adaptogenic: helps the body adapt to stress and exerts a normalizing effect upon bodily processes

Analgesic: reduces pain

Antacid: prevents or corrects acidity, especially in the stomach

Anticatarrhal: helps the body remove excess mucous

Antiemetic: prevents vomiting

Anti-inflammatory: controls or reduces inflammation

Antimicrobial: kills microorganisms or inhibits their growth

Antispasmodic: prevents or relieves spasms or convulsions

Aphrodisiac: stimulates sexual desire

Aromatic: stimulates the nervous and gastrointestinal systems through emissions of a pleasant and distinctive smell

Astringent: protects the skin and reduces bleeding from minor abrasions by prompting the contraction of body tissues

Bitter: stimulates digestion and aids in the elimination of toxins through a sharp, pungent taste or smell

Carminative: relieves flatulence

Demulcent: relieves irritation of the mucous membranes, particularly in the mouth and throat, by forming a protective film

Diaphoretic: induces perspiration

Diuretic: causes increased passing of urine

Emetic: induces vomiting

Emmenagogue: stimulates blood flow to the pelvic area or uterus, used especially to stimulate menstruation

Emollient: softens or soothes the skin

Expectorant: promotes the secretion of sputum by the air passages, used especially to treat coughs

Febrifuge: reduces fever

Hepatic: promotes liver function

Hypotensive: lowers blood pressure

Laxative: stimulates or facilitates evacuation of the bowels

Lymphatic: promotes lymphatic system function

Nervine: calms the nerves

Nootropic: enhances memory or other cognitive functions

Nutrient: provides nourishment essential for growth and the maintenance of life

Pectoral: strengthens the respiratory system

Rubefacient: produces redness of the skin by causing dilation of the capillaries and an increase in blood circulation

Sedative: induces sedation by reducing irritability or excitement

Stimulant: raises levels of physiological or nervous activity in the body

Styptic: helps stop bleeding when applied to a wound

Tonic: remedies imbalances in the body, prevents illness, and promotes longevity

Vasodilator: induces or initiates vasodilation by widening the interior cavity of blood vessels

Venotonic: promotes the structural integrity of the veins, helping to alleviate venous disorders and venous insufficiency

Vulnerary: helps heal wounds

RESOURCES

Learn more about herbs and herbal remedies:

American Botanical Council
www.herbalgram.org

American Herbalists Guild
www.americanherbalistsguild.com

Herb Research Foundation
www.herbs.org

Purchase quality herbs, ready-to-use preparations, and equipment:

Frontier Natural Products Co-op
www.frontiercoop.com

Gaia Herbs
www.gaiaherbs.com

Herb Pharm
www.herb-pharm.com

Mountain Rose Herbs
www.mountainroseherbs.com

Oregon's Wild Harvest
www.oregonswildharvest.com

Starwest Botanicals
www.starwest-botanicals.com

SUGGESTIONS FOR FURTHER READING

Adaptogens: Herbs for Strength, Stamina, and Stress Relief, by David Winston and Steven Maimes (Healing Arts Press, 2007).

Ancient Egyptian Medicine, by John F. Nunn (University of Oklahoma Press, 2002).

The Book of Herbal Wisdom: Using Plants as Medicines, by Matthew Wood (North Atlantic Books, 1997).

Culpeper's Complete Herbal: A Book of Natural Remedies for Ancient Ills, by Nicholas Culpeper (Wordsworth Editions, 1995).

The Green Pharmacy: New Discoveries in Herbal Remedies for Common Diseases and Conditions from the World's Foremost Authority on Healing Herbs, by James A. Duke (Rodale Press, 1997).

The Herbal or General History of Plants: The Complete 1633 Edition as Revised and Enlarged by Thomas Johnson, by John Gerard and Thomas Johnson (Dover Publications, 1975).

Let Thy Food Be Thy Medicine: Plants and Modern Medicine, by Kathleen L. Hefferon (Oxford University Press, 2012).

The Male Herbal: Health Care for Men & Boys, by James Green (Crossing Press, 1991).

Medicinal Plants in Folk Tradition: An Ethnobotany of Britain and Ireland, by David E. Allen and Gabrielle Hatfield (Timber Press, 2004).

A Modern Herbal: The Medicinal, Culinary, Cosmetic, and Economic Properties, Cultivation and Folklore of Herbs, Grasses, Fungi, Shrubs, & Trees with All Their Modern Scientific Uses, by Maud Grieve (Dover Publications, 1971).

National Geographic Guide to Medicinal Herbs: The World's Most Effective Healing Plants, by Rebecca L. Johnson, Steven Foster, Tieraona Low Dog, and David Kiefer (National Geographic, 2010).

Native American Ethnobotany, by Daniel E. Moerman (Timber Press, 1998).

Rosemary Gladstar's Medicinal Herbs: A Beginner's Guide, by Rosemary Gladstar (Storey Publishing, 2012).

Therapeutic Herb Manual: A Guide to the Safe and Effective Use of Liquid Herbal Extracts, by Ed Smith (Ed Smith, 1999).

ACKNOWLEDGMENTS

An extra special thanks goes to Matthew Valades, who is actually the best. I'm also grateful to my plant-loving friends and fellow herb nerds for all your encouragement and enthusiasm for this book. Thanks for sharing my excitement about the herbal wonders of the world and for getting me to talk about something else for a while, sometimes.

—Jean

With thanks to Mom and Dad, Jean, Katherine, and Ashley.

—Katie

INDEX